BS/MD Programs—
The Complete Guide

2016 EDITION

2016 EDITION
BS/MD Programs— The Complete Guide

GETTING INTO MEDICAL SCHOOL FROM HIGH SCHOOL

EXPANDED AND UP TO DATE

TODD A. JOHNSON

&

KELLEY ANNE JOHNSON

College Admissions Partners • Minnetonka, Minnesota

BS/MD Programs—The Complete Guide:
Getting into Medical School from High School

2016Edition

by Todd A. Johnson & Kelley Anne Johnson

Published by College Admissions Partners
601 Carlson Parkway Suite 1050
Minnetonka MN 55305
www.collegeadmissionspartners.com
todd@collegeadmissionspartners.com
952-449-5245

ISBN: 978-1-944911-00-3 trade paperback
       978-1-944911-01-0 e-book
ISSN: 2168-913X

Manufactured in the United States of America

Design and composition: www.dmargulis.com

To Susie and Caitlin,
for all of their support through the years.

Contents

Introduction: Why We Wrote This Book   1

1. What Are Early Acceptance Programs?   3

2. What It Takes to Be Competitive
   for BS/MD Programs   11

3. Finding the Right Program   25

4. The Application Essays   35

5. The Medical School Interview   51

6. Paying for Early Medical Programs   69

7. Other Issues Related to BS/MD Admissions   77

Appendix 1: BS/MD Programs by State   81

Appendix 2: BS/DO Programs by State   265

Index   279

Why We Wrote This Book

Every day, thousands of students dream of one day becoming a doctor. For most of these students, the pathway to medical school involves hard work in high school, so they can get into a good college. Once in college they must work hard to get good grades and eventually study for, and take, the Medical College Admission Test, the MCAT. Despite all of that hard work, many students will not be accepted into a medical school.

But, for the strongest and most dedicated students, for those students who have dreamed of becoming a doctor as long as they can remember, there is another option: early acceptance medical programs (EAMPs), commonly known as BS/MD programs. The EAMPs allow talented students to combine college and medical school into a guaranteed program leading to a medical degree.

In the past, there was limited information available to students seeking admission to these EAMPs. Students had to search for scattered bits of available information—and much of that information was incorrect.

We have helped hundreds of students get admitted into these highly competitive programs. The purpose of this book is to help students interested in EAMPs to understand all aspects of the available programs, including what it takes to be a serious candidate for admission. This book provides current information about which programs are available and the criteria needed for admission into the various programs. A website with up-to-date information about BS/MD programs is available at www.collegeadmissionspartners.com.

But, you want to know the details, so let's jump in.

1

What Are
Early Acceptance Programs?

EAMPs. Direct medical programs. BA/MD programs. BS/MD programs. BA/DO programs. These are just a few of the names that early acceptance medical programs go by. Let's first explore the similarities and differences between these types of early acceptance programs.

EAMP is a general term used to describe all of the various types of programs. All of the programs have one basic similarity: each program accepts high school students into both an undergraduate college and a medical school. If you maintain a specified grade point average during college, you have a guaranteed admission to medical school.

The only difference between BA/MD and BS/MD programs is the focus at the undergraduate college. A BA degree, or bachelor of arts, is used by colleges that require a broad educational background. As you work toward a BA degree, you typically take classes in a variety of subject areas during your first two years of college. These include science or math, humanities, and social sciences. In addition, many colleges that give a BA degree require that you show a certain level of competency in a foreign language. You concentrate on classes in your major during the last two years of college. The BA degree is by far the most common degree awarded by most colleges, even for science majors.

A BS degree, or bachelor of science, generally has a stronger focus on taking classes surrounding your major all four years of college. Most of these programs have few, if any, requirements for classes outside a specific major. While as a budding science major, you may think that only a BS degree is for you, be aware that most doctors have a BA degree. What degree you get is more a function of your personal desires and what school you attend than whether you will learn what you need to know to get into medical school. Some of the accelerated medical programs give a BS degree because you may only be in the undergraduate college for two or three years. During that time, you need to take primarily science courses since your undergraduate time is limited.

After finishing the undergraduate portion of a program and receiving the BA or BS, you then spend four years at the medical school and upon completion receive an MD or doctor of medicine degree.

BS/DO programs will be discussed in more detail in Chapter 3.

How Competitive Are These Programs?

The EAMPs are some of the most selective programs in college admissions. The most selective programs admit only one to two percent of the students who apply. Moreover, at the most selective colleges, the qualifications of the accepted students are extremely high. At Northwestern's Honors Program in Medical Education (HPME) the average SAT score for accepted students is over 2,300, and most of the students are in the top one percent of their high school classes. Their average SAT Math Level II score is 782 and the average SAT Chemistry subject test is 780.

Even those early acceptance programs that are "less" selective are extremely selective. The least selective programs still have very high average SAT scores and grade point averages. Make no mistake, no one is guaranteed acceptance into one of these programs regardless of their qualifications.

Many of the less selective early acceptance programs are located at public universities. Some of these public programs are available only to students of that state, and even those that are open to students from other states are much more selective for the out-of-state students. When you review the typical qualifications of the applicants for different programs, keep in mind whether the program is at a public or private university. If the program is public and you are out of state for that program, then you must have much higher qualifications to be competitive for admissions.

One last thought to keep in mind: no matter how strong your qualifications there are no guaranteed acceptances into these programs. Having good grades and test scores merely makes you competitive. But, even perfect grades and perfect test scores are not enough for acceptance. There are additional factors discussed later in the book, such as the quality of your essays and your interview, your experience in health care volunteering, and your interview, that help the medical schools determine who to admit into the programs.

How Long Do These Programs Last?

The normal length of education to become a doctor is eight years—four years of undergraduate college and four years of medical school. The early acceptance programs almost all include the standard four years for medical school.

But there is a difference among the programs on the length of the undergraduate education. Most early acceptance undergraduate programs last four years, which is the typical time to get a college degree. Some of these programs are accelerated, however. There are a few programs where you are at the undergraduate college for only two years and some where you are there three years. These accelerated programs grant the BA or BS degree after you have completed a portion of your medical school education. For example, a six-year EAMP will grant you a BS or BA degree after you have completed two years of college and two years of medical school. A seven-year program grants the undergraduate degree after three years of college and one year of medical school.

How Admissions Decisions Are Made

After you apply to an early acceptance program the undergraduate college's admissions department makes the first review of your qualifications. Because of the high minimum requirements to qualify for these programs, most students who apply will be accepted into the undergraduate colleges associated with the program. If you are accepted into the undergraduate college, your file is then sent to the medical school admissions committee for review. The medical school will evaluate your file and decide whether they would like to invite you for an interview at the medical school. Only if you are invited to interview will you continue to be considered for the program. The interview process is described in more detail in Chapter 5. Following the interview process, the medical school will determine which students to accept.

The Advantages of Early Acceptance Programs

There are a number of potential advantages to the student considering an early acceptance program. The obvious advantage is that if you are accepted into a program, you no longer have to worry about whether you will be accepted into a medical school. You are accepted.

Early acceptance can also ease your anxiety about the need to get very high grades during college. Most of the early acceptance programs specify minimum grades you must get, often a 3.5 GPA, during college. But the required grades are generally less than you would want to get if you had to worry about applying to medical school. This allows you to focus more on actually learning the subjects and less on the grades.

Students often feel they have more options in the types of courses they take during college while in an early acceptance program. Students trying to impress a medical admissions committee might not want to take classes in the humanities or social sciences. Instead they focus on hard science courses. Students involved with early acceptance programs can take the time to explore their interests outside the laboratory and often become better rounded students—and doctors—as a result.

A third potential benefit of some of the programs is the waiver of the requirement to take the Medical College Admission Test, the MCAT, before applying to medical school. Most students who take the MCAT spend a great deal of time preparing for the exam. If your program does not require this test, you have more time to be involved in other activities.

However, even if your program does not require early acceptance students to take the MCAT, there may be reasons to consider taking it. Some scholarships are available based on a student's MCAT score, and the failure to have a score will disqualify you from consideration for the scholarship. Certain combined degree programs such as MD/PhD programs also use the MCAT for admissions purposes. Finally, a few residency programs may consider the MCAT scores to determine placement into the residency.

A fourth benefit offered by many early acceptance programs is a range of enrichment activities for students in the program. As an example of these enrichment activities, let's take a look at Brown University's Program in Liberal Medical Education (PLME).

Brown has a Medicine in Action Program that offers undergraduates and medical students the opportunity to observe practicing physicians. They have several international exchange programs, including summer mini-courses in Germany as well as summer programs in China and Taiwan. In addition, Brown has the PLME Senate, a student organization that encourages early professional development among students involved in the program. Most accelerated programs have similar enrichment programs for their students.

A fifth benefit exists for those programs that last less than eight years. Obviously, in the accelerated BS/MD programs you will have fewer years of college and medical school. And that means fewer years of education to pay for.

The Disadvantages of Early Acceptance Programs

Despite all of the wonderful advantages associated with the EAMPs, they are not appropriate for all students. There are several potential disadvantages. Many of the early acceptance programs prohibit a student from applying to medical schools other than the one associated with the program. While this may not seem like much of a disadvantage, medical schools have personalities just like colleges. What is an appropriate medical school for one student may not be the most appropriate for another student. By committing to a particular medical school early, you may be sacrificing the option to attend another medical school that may be more appropriate.

A second disadvantage may exist for those programs that are shorter than the traditional four years of college. If you decide at some point during college that medicine is not what you wish to follow as a profession, there can be problems associated with graduation requirements.

However, the biggest potential disadvantage is a practical one. If you are academically competitive for early acceptance programs, you are likely to be a strong candidate for medical school even if you follow the traditional route of four years of college followed by application to medical school. Many of the early acceptance programs exist at colleges that may be weaker academically than you would traditionally consider. If you decide to follow a traditional path to medical school, you will likely attend a more academically competitive college. By attending a more academically competitive college, you will be a stronger candidate for a more competitive medical school. By going to a more competitive medical school, you may be in a better position to get the residency program you desire. The early acceptance programs limit your options. Whether that disadvantage outweighs the numerous advantages is for you to evaluate.

When to Start Preparing for BS/MD Programs

As we explain in Chapter 2, there are many things you have to do to be a competitive candidate for a BS/MD program. The earlier you start preparing, the better. Seventh and eighth grades are not too early to start thinking about the classes that you will take in high school. If you are able to take classes like algebra and geometry in these early grades you will be well positioned to take calculus in high school.

Exploring your extracurricular interests may also start at this stage, so that once you advance in high school you will be able to take leadership roles in your chosen activities. Volunteer efforts can also start at this stage. The strongest candidates will have several years of volunteer time at a single location rather than a smattering of volunteer activities here and there.

While an ideal candidate will have multiple years of consistent leadership and volunteer experience, it is never too late to enhance your experience and begin pursuing meaningful volunteer and extracurricular options.

Early Medical School Acceptance during College

Some colleges have programs that are named early acceptance programs but they are not the type of early acceptance being discussed by this book. These alternative early acceptance programs, commonly known as early assurance programs, allow students who are freshmen or sophomores at a particular college to apply to a program that allows early acceptance to an associated medical school if all of the required steps of the program are followed. These programs almost always require the student to take the MCAT and receive a certain minimum score to be admitted to the medical school. Because these programs do not provide early acceptance into the medical school as a high school student, we will not spend much time discussing them. However, they may be appropriate for some students. If you are not accepted into a true early acceptance program, you may wish to investigate the possibility of one of these programs as an alternative.

Some of the early assurance programs admit students into the program as incoming freshman although there is no guarantee of admissions to the medical school. St. Louis University is an example of such a program. Since admission to the medical school is not guaranteed, there is a somewhat higher admission rate into these programs. They can be a good option for students who are not as strong as the typical BS/MD applicant.

Chapter 2

What It Takes to Be Competitive for BS/MD Programs

The first question we are often asked is this: What does it take to be accepted into one of these EAMPs? Although there is nothing that will guarantee acceptance into an early acceptance program, there are a number of factors that programs look at in determining who to admit. This chapter will help you understand each of these factors and guide you in the quest to become the strongest possible candidate for an early acceptance program.

First, let's discuss the two factors that are required by many programs to even be considered: grades and test scores.

Grades

The most important factor for admission to an EAMP is your grades. The most common requirement is that you be in the top ten percent of your class to be a candidate for an early acceptance program. A few programs require you to be in the top five percent of your class. Some programs have, as an alternative requirement, that you have a certain grade point average to be considered for the program. A minimum 3.8 unweighted GPA is typical.

What happens if a program has a requirement that you be in the top ten percent of your class but your high school does not rank students? In our experience most early acceptance programs will ask for a minimum GPA under these circumstances, so as to not exclude students coming from high schools that don't rank.

A few early acceptance programs have no minimum GPA or class rank requirement for a student to be considered. These programs, however, tend to be the most selective programs. They have no minimum requirement because they don't want to exclude anyone from possible consideration. Don't be misled into thinking that you do not need high grades and class rank just because a program lists no minimums.

The range of grades that make you competitive for these programs varies. However, the minimum is generally an unweighted GPA of 3.5, and that is for state university programs that are seeking to encourage in-state students to apply for a program. To be the most competitive at the majority of the programs, you will need an unweighted GPA of 3.9 or higher and a class rank, if available, in the top one or two percent of your class.

Classes

Closely related to your grades are the classes you take to get those grades. BS/MD programs like to see students who have challenged themselves in their classes. Ideally, students will take four years of each of the five core subjects: math, science, English, social studies, and a single foreign language. While few colleges require this type of course load, most of the students that you will competing against will have most, if not all, of these classes.

Some BS/MD programs have specific requirements on which classes students must take to be able to apply. Most commonly they require a year each of biology, chemistry, and physics; but many colleges also require four years of English and four years of math. And while few colleges require calculus, we cannot recall any of our students being admitted to a BS/MD program without having calculus. Whether it is

AB or BC doesn't seem to make any difference as long as you have one of those courses or the equivalent.

So, besides asking that you take all of the core subjects, what do BS/MD programs mean when they talk about challenging classes. Usually it means that students will have taken an appropriate number of AP or IB classes, particularly in the sciences and math. While you don't need to take every AP class your school offers, you do need to take a significant number. Our typical BS/MD students have taken between six and ten AP classes while in high school.

Does it make any difference if a student takes AP classes versus IB classes? In our experience, we have not seen any difference in admissions rates for one program versus the other. We can say that admissions officers are impressed with students taking IB classes who get a full IB diploma.

Test Scores

The second factor required for early acceptance programs is a strong standardized test score. Most programs require a minimum SAT score between 1,350 and 1,450 exclusive of the writing sub-score. Again, these are minimum requirements. To be the most competitive you should have a score over 2,250 on the SAT or 34 on the ACT.

While the majority of colleges super-score the SAT for general admissions, early acceptance programs do not typically super-score the SAT for admissions to these programs. Super-scoring means taking the highest subsection score from multiple test dates and combining the highest scores to make a super-score. For example, suppose you take the SAT twice and the first time receive a 600 verbal and 700 math. The second time you take the SAT you receive a 700 verbal and 620 math. Although the highest score from one sitting is the 1,320 from the second test, a college that super-scores will combine the 700 verbal from the second test with the 700 math from the first test to give a super-score of 1,400.

Some programs also state a minimum ACT score for students taking that test. Most commonly, the minimum ACT score is a 30 composite score. Those programs that don't state a minimum ACT convert an ACT score into an SAT score. A few programs prefer to see either the SAT or the ACT test, and they will tell you their preference.

In addition to the SAT or ACT tests, many of the programs also want to see two SAT subject test scores. Some programs tell you specifically what subject test scores they would like to see; but if they don't say, the best option is to take the Math II subject test and either the Chemistry or the Biology subject test. Again, to be most competitive you want to score greater than 700 on each of the subject tests.

All right, you say you have great grades and your tests scores are wonderful, but rarely will these factors alone lead to acceptance into a BS/MD program. A myriad of other factors are considered for admissions into early acceptance programs.

Research Experience

Most competitive students applying to early acceptance programs have some type of scientific research experience, most commonly in the fields of biology or chemistry. This is often as a result of a research opportunity at a university that the student participated in during one of their summers but may also have occurred during the school year. While there are no specific requirements that an applicant have research experience, the early acceptance programs look very favorably on this type of experience, as it further confirms your interest in a scientific field. Contrary to what many people may think, this research does not need to be related to a medical field.

A common question we are asked is, How does a student find a research opportunity? There are two basic ways this occurs. The first option, which is often preferable, is to have a student find their own research at a college or university that is close to where they live. Many students are able to do this by investigating the professors at the university to see who is doing research that the student finds interesting. The student can then contact the professor and ask to be part of the research team, usually during the summer before junior or senior year. To have the best chance of having a professor agree to this, you will need to make it clear that you are interested in research and that you are a strong student in math and science. You should first contact the professor in the January before the summer you wish to do the research.

The second option to get research is usually simpler. There are many colleges around the country that sponsor summer research opportunities for high school students. Some of them are competitive and require an application, and these generally are available in January and February. These programs also charge for the student to participate, and they can be quite expensive.

The reason we prefer the first option, aside from the obvious cost savings, is that it shows a certain level of maturity for a student to contact a college professor and arrange their own research opportunity. And as we will see later in this chapter, maturity is a major factor in admissions for BS/MD programs.

Volunteer Activities

Most colleges like to see applicants who have volunteered their time to help others. This is particularly true for early acceptance programs, because they are looking for students who show compassion. There are few better ways to show compassion than by volunteering. Ideally, some of this volunteer effort should occur in a health-related setting such as a clinic, hospital, or nursing home.

We have had many students who volunteered in nursing homes. Nursing homes are often a good place to volunteer, because they don't typically have many restrictions on who can volunteer or what they do. Some of our students have gone to the nursing homes on a regular basis to visit with residents. Others went to play musical instruments, read books to those who are vision-impaired, or help with feeding residents.

Nursing homes are not the only place you can volunteer. Many hospitals will gladly work with a student who wishes to volunteer. This often involves helping in a gift shop or helping direct people who are visiting the hospital. While this type of volunteering is good, it is best if you can be in a position of interacting with patients. For instance, many of our students have had the opportunity to volunteer in an emergency room or an outpatient surgery area. This type of volunteering, however, can be hard to come by in a hospital. That is why the nursing home setting can be more useful.

There is no minimum number of volunteer hours needed, and it is not necessary to record the number of hours you have as a volunteer. However, it is obvious to anyone if you have not been serious about showing true compassion. This is not about fulfilling a requirement. This is about really showing that you are engaged and you care. We generally advise students that the longer a particular volunteer effort has been going on, the greater the weight it will be given. Ideally, you will have volunteered for more than one year at one or more facilities. You do not need to devote all of your time to volunteering. One or two hours a week, if done consistently during the year, is sufficient.

Physician Shadowing

Early acceptance programs also like to see that a student has performed some type of physician shadowing. Early acceptance programs want to admit only those students who are truly committed to becoming a physician. Many students start college declaring their intent to become physicians; yet the majority of these students change their plans along the way for various reasons. Early acceptance programs want to minimize the number of students who change their minds about becoming physicians. One of the ways you can convince the programs you are serious about becoming a physician is to show that you have followed one or more doctors around to see what their typical day is like.

Many doctors are happy to have a student shadow them if you explain that you are committed to attending medical school and want to experience what their actual work is like. Many students follow a doctor around in a clinical setting, but many also are able to make hospital rounds and even observe surgery. It does not matter what type of physician you shadow; but if you think you might have a particular interest in one field of medicine, then see if you can shadow a physician who specializes in that field. There is no minimum amount of time you have to do the shadowing, but we usually recommend that students try to spend at least 40 hours shadowing a physician. If you wish to do more than this, it is fine; but volunteering is usually a better way to spend your time after 40 hours.

Extracurricular Activities

Another significant factor in the admissions process for early acceptance programs is the evaluation of the student's extracurricular activities.

There should be a focus on leadership in your activities during junior and senior year. Early acceptance programs are not interested in students who join many different activities but do not seriously pursue any of them. Rather, a long-term commitment to the activity is what these programs are looking for. Ideally, you should be involved in those activities that interest you the most; and it is best if you have some leadership experience in those activities.

People often ask what the best extracurricular activity is, but the reality is that there is no one right activity. Colleges want to see you involved in activities that are of particular interest to you. These may be activities related to school, but they can just as easily be activities outside of school. The focus of these activities, however, is often different for early acceptance students than for students applying only to highly selective colleges.

The most selective colleges are looking for students who are specialists in a particular activity. These are the students who have focused all of their interest on a select few activities—the student whose life revolves around the clarinet, the tennis court, or the chemistry lab.

Early acceptance programs, on the other hand, tend to favor students who have a somewhat broader background. You might be involved in the band, student government, and science Olympiad all at the same time. As long as you have been seriously involved in each of your activities, you will be a strong candidate. What does it mean to be seriously involved? It means that you have been involved with the activity through most, if not all, of your high school career, devoting substantial time to the activity and ideally achieving a leadership position of some sort.

One difference with the extracurricular activities for those students interested in early acceptance programs is the importance of a focus on health-related activities. This might include involvement in, or the founding of, a chapter of Future Doctors of America, involvement with science Olympiad, or other activities that have some relationship with the health care field.

Many students, in completing the list of extracurricular activities on the application, want to list every activity they have been involved in since they were young. This is not a good idea. You want to focus your extracurricular activities on those that show your interest in health care, that highlight your leadership, or that reflect those activities that you have been seriously involved with. That one hour that you rang the bell for the Salvation Army should not be listed. Although it is a volunteer activity, listing this type of limited involvement activity either looks like you don't have enough serious volunteer activities or you are shallow and pandering. Neither is the impression you want to give a medical school admissions committee.

There are two basic ways to provide the colleges with information about your extracurricular activities. The most common is through the activity list of the Common Application. The Common Application provides room for ten activities. For each activity you can list the years devoted to the activity, the number of hours per week, the number of weeks per year, your position in the activity, and a brief statement of what the activity involves. You can also indicate if this is an activity that you intend to continue in college.

There are several advantages to using the activity list of the Common Application as your only list of activities. First, it is simple. You don't have to worry about how to structure a list of activities; the list is ready for you to complete. And because of the limited space available, you have to choose only those activities that are most important to you and to be succinct in describing each activity.

The second advantage is that the activity list on the Common Application makes it simple for the college admissions reader to review all of your activities at a glance. Given that a typical application only gets fifteen to twenty minutes of review for the entire application, having a convenient list of the most important activities is helpful. For most students we recommend that they use the Common Application list for activities as their exclusive list.

However, there is another option that is appropriate for some students. For some students with a large number of strong activities, the supplemental activities résumé may be appropriate. This supplemental résumé is a supplement to the activities list on the Common Application. This supplemental résumé should only include activities not already included on the Common Application list of activities. The major advantage of the supplemental résumé is that it lets you provide greater detail about specific activities and it allows the listing of a greater number of activities. Many counselors encourage all of their students to submit a supplemental résumé rather than use the application list of the Common Application. While this may seem like a wise idea, we believe that it actually works to the disadvantage of many students.

There are several issues that should be considered by the student who is considering using a supplemental résumé. First, remember that a college admissions officer has limited time to look at the entire application. As mentioned earlier, fifteen to twenty minutes is typical for the time to review an application.

Now imagine that you have just submitted a three-page résumé of activities. If the admissions officer looks at your entire résumé, they will have that much less time to review the rest of your application, including your grades, classes, test scores, and essays. What typically happens in these situations is that the admissions officer spends the usual amount of time looking at your grades, classes, test scores, and essays. They then take the limited amount of time they have left to scan over your résumé. If the résumé is too detailed, or too long, the admissions officer may miss some of your activities just because they don't have time to review each application in that kind of detail. You may also annoy the admissions reader because they are trying to be fair to everyone whose application they have to read. If they feel that they have to spend more time on your résumé than on some other student's, it will generally not help, and may hurt, your chance of admissions.

The second factor to consider if you are thinking about doing a supplemental résumé is whether you really have enough activities to justify such a résumé. There are some students that have an incredible amount of serious extracurricular activities that cannot be accounted for by the Common Application. But this is the unusual circumstance.

The third factor to consider is how it looks on your application that you are not able to write succinctly to describe your activities. Colleges using the Common Application do so intentionally to make sure that they get the information they require. Colleges are not pushing the Common Application to increase the number of listings for activities or to give more space for the description of the activities. That is because they know that for most students, the allowed space is sufficient to list the most important activities.

If you really believe you have too many activities for the Common Application, or that you need to provide more detail on your activities than the space on the Common Application allows, try to limit the supplemental résumé to one page of single spaced type. Follow the same format as the Common Application so that similar information is included in your supplemental résumé. Choose an ordinary serif typeface that is easily read on paper or computer monitor, such as Century Schoolbook (what you are reading now) or Garamond, in 12-point size. If space is tight, you can use Times New Roman, instead. Do not try to demonstrate your creativity by selecting a script font or an informal font such as Comic Sans. Doing so will detract from the image you are presenting.

The Common Application provides a space for you to provide any additional information that you would like the college to know about. This is the space that can be used to expand on your activities using a supplemental résumé, if you choose to include one.

Despite our reservations about using résumés in the application, there are times when it is helpful to have a short, one- or two-page résumé. When you interview with either a college or medical school, it can sometimes be helpful to have a résumé to help your interviewer know what activities you have been involved with.

There are also a few medical schools that specifically ask for a résumé, so having one available can be helpful. Just remember, longer is not better when it comes to a résumé.

Recommendations

Most EAMPs require two teacher recommendations and a counselor recommendation. For most colleges, recommendations have little influence on the admissions decisions. However, in programs that are extremely competitive, such as EAMPs, any small advantage is important.

To get the best recommendations from your teachers and counselor you want to make sure that they have information on all of your background. One easy way is to provide them with a résumé. Remember that résumé you wanted to put together for the application? Use that résumé instead to provide complete information to your recommenders.

Ideally, the recommendation will focus on those issues that are important to an EAMP. Comments about your maturity, your intellectual curiosity, your helpfulness in the classroom, your volunteer activities, and your leadership are all helpful. You want to be sure that your recommenders are aware of your commitment to attending medical school, and you may ask them to comment on this focus. Familiarity of the recommender with any extended health care volunteer activities would also be helpful.

Students often do not have a strong relationship with their high school counselor because the counselor has a large number of students to work with. If that is true of your counselor, you need to make every effort to get to know your counselor as well as possible before they need to write your recommendation. Colleges understand that high schools often have high counselor-to-student ratios so will not penalize you if you don't get a detailed recommendation from your counselor. But, if you can get a good recommendation from your counselor, it is one more small step in helping the application reader understand who you are.

Students often wish to provide more recommendations than are asked for by the college. It is the rare situation when it is appropriate to send additional recommendation letters. Colleges ask for the information that they think they need to make a reasoned decision. If they wanted more recommendations, they would ask for them. The only time it is appropriate to provide an additional recommendation is if that recommender can offer a perspective on an important aspect of your background that is not addressed elsewhere in the application.

Final Thoughts

Colleges and in particular medical schools are not just looking for the brightest students. Yes, you need the grades and test scores to be eligible for BS/MD programs. But good grades and test scores alone are not enough to impress BS/MD programs. You also need to show that you have the passion to be a physician and the compassion to be a good doctor. You need to show that you have the maturity to handle the pressure of medical school and the life of a physician. You must communicate that you are conscientious but also personable.

How do you show that you have these personality characteristics? This information should come out in all aspects of your application. Your college and medical school essays, your activity list, your recommendations, and your interview all are opportunities to communicate who you are beyond your transcript. As you proceed through your application to a BS/MD program do not lose sight of who you are and how you might communicate that to the programs.

Chapter 3

Finding the Right Program

Now that you know what you have to do to be competitive for an EAMP, let's look at the various choices you have to make to ensure you find the right program for your needs.

What Is the Length of the Early Acceptance Program?

As we have already seen, these programs can last six, seven, or eight years. Six-year programs are probably the least common, while eight-year programs are the most common. The advantage to the six-year programs is you can finish a traditional eight-year program in only six years. You do this by focusing on the required basic science classes during the first two years of undergraduate education. You then start the medical school portion of your training and are awarded your undergraduate degree after the first two years of medical school.

What you lose from a shortened program is the ability to take classes outside of the basic sciences, since you have only two years of undergraduate education. Doctors need to understand the basic sciences, and all early acceptance programs preserve that need. However, being a good doctor involves much more than just understanding the science.

Having a background in the humanities can give a doctor a broader base of knowledge when dealing with patients. The study of subjects such as sociology, psychology, and anthropology may help you understand the patient from a personal and cultural standpoint. Having additional years of undergraduate college also allows you to study a foreign language in more detail. Having more years of college allows students to become better communicators, and being able to talk with patients is a vital part of most physicians' lives.

Does the Program Exempt Students from Taking the MCAT?

The Medical College Admission Test (MCAT) often creates a great deal of anxiety among students interested in attending medical school. At most medical schools, the results of the MCAT is second only to a student's college grades in determining who will be admitted to medical school. The MCAT generally requires a great deal of time and preparation if a student is to score well.

Many of the early acceptance programs do not require that you take the MCAT before starting the medical school portion of your education. The opportunity to avoid the MCAT is a major motivation for many students to consider early acceptance programs. If you are concerned about taking the MCAT, you may want to focus on programs that do not require the submission of the test. Even if you are a strong test taker, you may wish to avoid the MCAT so that you can use the time normally taken in test preparation for other purposes. In fact, avoiding the MCAT could give you enough time to take another class or become more involved in a particular activity.

There are a number of early acceptance programs, however, that do require the MCAT. Among those programs, some require a minimum MCAT score and others have no set minimum score. If the program that you are considering is one that requires the MCAT be taken, check to see if there is any required minimum score. If not, much of the pressure associated with the MCAT is reduced even if you need to take the test.

If the program you are interested in has a minimum score, look to see how high that score is. If it is a relatively low score, you may not need to devote a great deal of time to the MCAT. However, some programs have a relatively high minimum MCAT score. The early acceptance program between Lehigh University and Drexel University College of Medicine has a minimum MCAT score of 31. A score of 31 on the MCAT is the average MCAT score of students admitted to the Drexel College of Medicine through the regular admissions route. Thus, at a program like the Lehigh–Drexel program, a student in the early acceptance program would need to study more for the MCAT than would a student applying to Drexel University College of Medicine.

How Clinical Training Is Addressed by the Medical School

The first two years of medical school are typically devoted to an in-depth look at the systems of the body. This is primarily an academic approach in the classroom or the laboratory. In the last two years of medical school, the students go to various clinical sites that allow them to actually start interacting with patients.

There is a current trend among some medical schools to better integrate clinical training and classroom training. Some programs provide clinical experiences in the first year, but the extent of early clinical experiences varies by program. If you are interested in having clinical experiences all four years of medical school, you will want to ask the medical school how they handle clinical training.

The other question you should investigate is what clinical options are available during medical school. Ideally, the clinical sites are in large hospitals or clinical settings where you can see a variety of medical problems. The broader the types of patients and problems you see, the more likely you will have the experience to do well on the national medical tests required during medical school. If a clinical setting has little variety in the types of patients seen, you will be at a disadvantage when taking the national exams.

What Is the Medical School's USMLE Pass Rate?

This question is closely related to the one we just discussed regarding the available clinical sites. Medical students must take a series of exams known in general as the United States Medical Licensing Exam (USMLE). There are several parts to this exam, taken at various times during a medical student's education. Part 1 of the exam is taken after the first two years of medical school. This part of the exam tests your understanding of the basic scientific concepts necessary to practice medicine.

Part 2 of the exam is typically taken during the fourth year of medical school. Part 2 itself is divided into two tests. The first exam of Part 2, CK, tests the clinical knowledge you have acquired. The second part of the exam, CS, tests the clinical skills you have acquired as you near completion of your formal education. It is in Part 2 of the exam that the program's clinical sites can play an important role.

Obviously, you wish to see pass rates as close to one hundred percent as possible on both portions of this exam for each early acceptance program you are considering. In 2013, the pass rate for Part 1 examinations from students attending a US or Canadian MD program was ninety-five percent. For students attending a DO program, the average pass rate was ninety-four percent.

The pass rate that year for Part 2 CK examinations for students attending a US or Canadian MD program was ninety-seven percent. For those students in a DO program, the pass rate was ninety-six percent. For Part 2 CS exams, the pass rate was ninety-seven percent for US or Canadian MD programs and eighty-nine percent for DO programs.

If the program you are considering has pass rates on either section of the USMLE substantially lower than the national average, you should ask pointed questions on why they have a lower pass rate.

How Effective Is the Medical School at Matching Students into One of the Student's Top Three Residency Choices?

Once you finish medical school, the next step in your education is the residency, where you spend several years working on your particular specialty. The process of determining where the residency will occur is known as a match program. Students specify their preferences for where they would like to do their residency, and residency programs then look at the list of students who wish to attend their program to see which students they will accept. There are a variety of factors that go into the decision of who will be offered a residency at a particular program. Common factors include the strength of the medical school, the grades earned by the student, and the scores the student received on their USMLE exam.

As a student, your biggest concern is getting into one of your top options for a residency program. At times, even strong students from strong medical schools will not match one of their top programs. If few of the medical school's students match their top options for a residency program, you will want to ask questions.

What Are the Requirements of the Undergraduate Portion of the Program?

Although each of these programs guarantees admission to a medical school upon completion of the undergraduate study, there are requirements during the undergraduate years that must be met. You need to understand what those requirements are for each of the program you are interested in. Usually you need to maintain a minimum overall grade point average as well as a minimum grade point average for science and math courses. Most commonly this is a 3.5 GPA. Some can be higher. For instance, Washington University's University Scholar in Medicine program requires that students maintain a 3.8 GPA. If you have a high school GPA of 4.0, you may not think that sounds bad. But be aware that getting a GPA of 3.8 at a competitive college is not as easy as it may sound.

Other common requirements for students in these programs include occasional evaluations of your work by members of the BS/MD committee, attending scheduled meetings related to the program, and participation in volunteer service projects.

What Is the Completion Rate for the Program?

You will want to ask the early acceptance programs how many of the students who start the program actually finish. There are many reasons why someone might decide not to complete an early acceptance program. Some students may decide that their interest in medicine is not as strong as they thought it was before starting the program, while others find that academically, the program is more difficult than they thought. You should not be concerned if a few people leave the program each year.

However, if a large percentage of people leave the program, you need to ask further questions to find out why people are leaving the program. The biggest concern is if people are not finishing the program because they were not able to meet the minimum grade requirements. You should ask how many people leave the program because they were not successful academically. This might be because students did not have adequate preparation in high school, or it may be that there are problems getting the required grades in a required class. The University of Alabama Birmingham has stated that fifteen percent of students admitted to their program fail out and fifty percent are on probation at some time during their undergraduate years. You will want to know that same information for the programs you are considering.

What Ability Do You Have to Attend Other Colleges or Medical Schools?

Just as not all colleges are appropriate for all students, not all medical schools are appropriate for all students. You may find that the focus of the medical school associated with the early acceptance program is not consistent with your focus. Or you may find that the teaching style at the medical school makes it difficult for you to learn the necessary lessons. If you find, for whatever reason, that the medical school just is not appropriate, what opportunities do you have to apply to another medical school?

Most programs specify that you lose your guaranteed spot at the medical school if you decide to apply to other medical schools. You would still have the option to be considered as a regular applicant, but you would have no advantages over other candidates. If you think you may wish to have the option to apply to other medical schools, you should only consider those programs that allow you to maintain your guaranteed spot even while applying to other medical schools.

If you decide that the undergraduate college is not appropriate you will want to know how easy it is to transfer to another college. The sequence of courses with some programs may make it difficult to transfer to another college. This is particularly true for the six- and seven-year accelerated programs.

What Happens if You Decide Not to Attend Medical School

No one goes into an EAMP with the thought they might change their mind and decide not to attend medical school.

But, every year, certain students decide that medical school is just not right for them. Even if you are sure that this will never happen to you, it only takes a few questions to find out what will happen if you have a change of heart.

In most programs, deciding not to pursue medical school is not a problem, because you would just continue on as a regular college student at the undergraduate college. However, there can be problems if you are on an accelerated program that lasts six or seven years. Remember that for the accelerated programs, the reduced time is at the undergraduate level. What happens if you are in a six-year program and, in the first year of medical school, you decide medicine just isn't for you? You will not receive your undergraduate degree until you finish your second year of medical school. But, if you don't finish two years of medical school, what do you need to do to finish your undergraduate degree?

Remember that you are choosing not only an undergraduate college but also a medical school when you apply to an early acceptance program. For the best fit you need to make sure you are applying not only to the best college for your needs but also to the best medical school for your needs.

If you have more questions about a particular program, you should talk to people involved in the program, including professors at the undergraduate and medical school level. If there are concerns about the number of people who leave the program, you should ask about this issue. You may also wish to talk with students who are currently in the program to get their thoughts on how well the program is run and whether they feel prepared to advance to the medical school or take the USMLE exams. You should be able to ask the program to give you the contact information for current students who can answer your questions.

Should You Consider a BS/DO Program

To understand the BA/DO programs, we need a quick history lesson. The DO degree, or the doctor of osteopathy, developed in the late 1800s as an alternative to the MD degree. Doctors with a DO degree get basically the same training as MDs but with additional training in manipulation of the bones. At this point all states recognize the MD and DO degree as both qualified to practice medicine. The American Medical Association allows both types of doctors to become members.

The BA/DO programs are at undergraduate colleges associated with an osteopathic medical college. Otherwise, they are very similar to BA/MD programs. There are BS/DO programs just as there are BS/MD programs. This book deals primarily with those programs associated with medical schools leading to the MD degree, since these are much more common programs. However, we do want to highlight a few of the differences.

The BS/DO programs do tend to be somewhat less competitive, so students with slightly lower grades and test scores may be competitive for a BS/DO program even though they would not be competitive for a BS/MD program.

To be considered for a BS/DO program students should generally have at least a 1,200 critical reading and math score or a 27 ACT. A high school unweighted GPA of 3.5 or better would normally be expected. Just like BS/MD programs, they also want to see health care–related volunteering, research, maturity, and leadership. Doctor shadowing is also expected, but, if you are considering applying to BS/DO programs, you should shadow a physician with a DO degree and understand the difference in philosophies of the two types of medicine.

Understanding this difference is critical for BS/DO interviews, and it is not uncommon to be asked why you are interested in BS/DO programs instead of BS/MD programs. Failure to have an answer will most likely keep you from being considered.

Students with a DO degree are eligible for every medical specialty and the vast majority of residency programs. There are some residency programs just for DO students.

Chapter 4

The Application Essays

Most students applying to early acceptance programs are very high achieving students with high grades and high test scores. So how do colleges distinguish between all of these strong students? One way is by reviewing the application essays. In this chapter we will look in more detail at the various essays that may be required in the application for early acceptance programs. First, let's examine the essays required for the undergraduate portion of the application.

Undergraduate College Application Essay

Colleges use the undergraduate application essays for several purposes. First, they want to see how well you can write. The ability to write well is critical in college regardless of your major. Reviewing your application essays is one of the ways colleges evaluate your ability to write well. They also look at your grades in English classes and your score on the writing section of the SAT or ACT as further verification of your ability to write.

A second purpose of the application essay is to provide the application reader some insight into the applicant as a person beyond the grades and test scores. We will discuss what to write about in a little bit, but understand for now that you do not want to be discussing grades and test scores in your application essay. This is your chance to showcase something else about why you are a strong applicant.

Before we start talking about the essays, just a few words on the mechanics of writing an essay. You do not need to title your essay unless you think that a title will add something to the essay itself. In most cases, the writing should be able to convey your story without a title. If it does not, then you need to work some more on the essay.

Unless the instructions specifically ask for single line spacing, use double line spacing, with one-inch page margins, as this improves readability. Use the same typeface and size you chose for the Common Application, such as 12-point Garamond or Century Schoolbook (or another ordinary-looking serif typeface). You want the reader to focus on what you wrote, not on your taste in exotic fonts.

Enough of the mechanics. Let's talk about the essays themselves.

Common Application Essays

Most of the early admissions medical programs (EAMPs) use the Common Application for the application to the undergraduate college. The Common Application has the personal essay, which allows you to show the application reader how well you write and to reveal a little more about the person behind the application. This has a minimum length of 250 words and a maximum length of 650 words.

Be aware, however, that the essay is a very personal piece of writing, and focusing too much on length can make for a bad essay. We have seen wonderful essays that barely made the 250 word limit. Write to communicate what you wish to communicate, and stop writing. If it is over 650 words, then review the essay to focus on the most important elements while not exceeding 650 words.

Your first job with the personal essay is to decide which prompt you wish to write about. The Common Application this past year had five standard essay prompts, which are listed here.

1. Some students have a background or story that is so
    central to their identity that they believe their appli-
    cation would be incomplete without it. If this sounds
    like you, then please share your story.
2. Recount an incident or time when you experienced
    failure. How did it affect you, and what lessons did
    you learn?
3. Reflect on a time when you challenged a belief or idea.
    What prompted you to act? Would you make the same
    decision again?
4. Describe a place or environment where you are per-
    fectly content. What do you do or experience there,
    and why is it meaningful to you?
5. Discuss an accomplishment or event, formal or infor-
    mal, that marked your transition from childhood to
    adulthood within your culture, community, or family.

Prompts © The Common Application. Used with permission.

You can use the above prompts to give you some idea of the
types of questions that might be asked. One choice is not
better than another. Read through each of the prompts and
see if there is any one that is particularly appealing to you.

In brainstorming for ideas to write about, you want to
keep in mind that the application reader is looking for a little
insight into who you are beyond grades and test scores. They
have your transcript, your official test scores, and a list of
activities in the application. Do not repeat any of that information. You want to communicate one small part of who you
are or something in your life that has influenced who you
are or how you think. The biggest mistake most students
make in writing the personal essay is to tackle too broad a
topic. The purpose of this book is not to go into great detail
about writing the college application. However, because of
the importance of the application, We would strongly urge
you to consider looking at one of the books that discuss writ-

ing the college application essay. One of the best is Harry Bauld's book, *On Writing the College Application Essay.*

While guiding you through the college application essay is not the goal of this book, improving your standing as an applicant to an early admissions medical program is. So how do you write the personal essay to enhance your application to such programs? Always keep in mind what qualities the colleges and medical colleges are looking for in successful applicants. They are looking for students with leadership abilities, with maturity, and with compassion. You may not be able to write an essay that covers each of these topics, but you can focus your essay on one of them. Which one does not matter, although we would lean toward an essay that shows you have true compassion for others.

While this may seem an ideal place to write an essay on your passion for becoming a physician, this is one topic that should be avoided in this essay. All of the BS/MD programs will ask about your interest in becoming a physician in a supplemental essay. If you answer that question in the common application, you will not have much left when it comes time to respond to the question on the supplements.

In the past the Common Application also had a short answer section where the prompt was "Please briefly elaborate on one of your extracurricular activities or work experiences in the space below or on an attached sheet (150 words or fewer)." Although this essay is no longer part of the common application, many colleges are asking this question as one of their supplement questions. It does not matter which activity you choose to write about, but it should be one that strengthens your résumé for early acceptance programs. Writing about your involvement with the baseball team may make a good short essay, but something that relates to your involvement with an activity that shows compassion or a health-related activity would be even better.

One additional caution when writing the Common Application essay. While it is fine to be self-assured, you want to make sure that you do not come across as bragging about yourself. Medical schools do not want students who are self-impressed. In your essay don't talk about how everyone looks up to you or how you are well known for your volunteer activities. You want to present a more humble approach in your essays. Let your recommendations talk about what a great student you are that everyone looks up to.

The Common Application has another writing section that can be used. The prompt says, "Please provide an answer below if you wish to provide details of circumstances or qualifications not reflected in the application." This is yet another opportunity to communicate your unique strength and why you should be considered a strong candidate for an early acceptance program. You have 650 words in which to provide your response, and this is a fairly significant space. You do not want to repeat anything that has already been discussed in the rest of the application. But, as an example, if you have done significant research, this is a good place to put an abstract of your research. Or, if you have more activities than can fit on the common application list of activities, this is a place for those. You do not need to use the entire 650 words if you can answer in less space. Remember that your entire application will be read in a limited period, so you do not want to waste space.

The Common Application provides two places to discuss some aspect of who you are. Each of the sections should discuss a different aspect of your life. You do not want to talk about the humanitarian club you founded in both sections, for instance. This makes it sound as if you don't have the depth of involvement to be a serious candidate for early acceptance.

If that was not enough space to talk about yourself and your involvement with different activities, most colleges also have supplemental essays to the Common Application. Most of the college-specific essays fall into one of two types: "What will you add to our community" questions; and "Why are you interested in our college" questions. Rice University, for instance, asks: "The quality of Rice's academic life and the Residential College System are heavily influenced by the unique life experiences and cultural traditions each student brings. What perspective do you feel that you will contribute to life at Rice?" This question from Rice makes it clear that they are not seeking everyday, boring students. They want students who are interesting and engaged in the world around them. If you have health care experiences in a foreign country, this would be a great time to write about that experience. It answers the question about what makes you interesting, and it once again ties in your interest in the health care field.

Northwestern University's essay question focuses more on why you wish to attend that college but again leaves room for you to distinguish yourself from other applicants: "What are the unique qualities of Northwestern— and of the specific undergraduate school to which you are applying— that make you want to attend the University? In what ways do you hope to take advantage of the qualities you have identified?" When answering a question about why you wish to attend a particular college, you should be specific. Look at your answer after you have it written. If you can substitute the name of another college in place of the college you are applying to, the answer is too generic.

Look at the mission statement of each college that asks for an essay like this. The college's mission statement tells you how the college views itself and how they believe that they are different from other colleges. Another idea is to look at the departmental webpage of the major you are considering. Most colleges give biographies of the faculty in that department. If you find a particular professor that is working on something that is of interest to you, reference your interest in that professor's work in your essay.

If you are applying to an EAMP that does not use the Common Application, you may have less work to do for the initial college application. The University of Missouri at Kansas City early acceptance program, for instance, has no essay requirement for the undergraduate application. Some of the other non–Common Application colleges do have essay requirements, but they tend to be fairly general questions that you may be able to use the Common Application personal essay for.

Medical School Essays

You have submitted your undergraduate application; and now, if you are lucky, you will be asked to answer some essays from the medical school. The undergraduate essays are used primarily to see how well you write and to give the admissions committee some further insight into who you are. The medical school admissions committee is looking at your essays for this same information. But the people reviewing medical school essays are looking at much more. Depending on the particular question, the medical essays tend to fall into one of the following four categories.

- Motivation
- Commitment
- Diligence
- Maturity

Motivation

The first type of medical school question is one that looks at your motivation for becoming a doctor. Are you interested in the healing art of medicine, or is your focus on becoming rich and successful? Hint: the right answer is not "becoming rich and successful." While this may seem obvious, we often see students talk about the prestige of becoming a doctor. Yes, being a doctor can be prestigious. But if that is your focus, then the EAMPs are not going to be impressed.

So, how do you show what your motivation is? Discuss something that has occurred in your life that provides a personal touch. Maybe you were injured as a child and were inspired by the care provided by your doctors. Maybe you watched a relative suffer a debilitating illness and you were impressed by the compassion of the doctors who treated your relative.

You may also show your motivation through the activities in which you have been involved. Are you founder of a group that provides regular visits to nursing home residents? Have you been involved in an activity for several years where the only compensation is the good feeling you receive? These are the sorts of experiences that medical schools are looking for in strong applicants to early admissions programs. Depth of involvement in a particular activity is much more important here than the number of activities you may have been involved in.

Commitment

The second type of medical school essay tries to confirm that you are serious about becoming a doctor and will continue through the early acceptance program if you are accepted. Many students start college planning to go to medical school but never finish the necessarily coursework. This occurs for many reasons including the inability of the student to handle the work but also a lack of motivation when the hard work needs to be done. Medical schools do not want to waste an acceptance on a student who may not be serious about becoming a doctor. In fact, the basic academic requirements to even apply to early acceptance programs are designed to weed out those students who may not be able to handle the academic rigors of the coursework.

Your answers to the essay questions are another way for the medical admissions committee to get a feel for how serious you are about becoming a doctor. There are a number of ways to show the depth of your commitment to becoming a doctor. Most of these we have already discussed, such as doctor shadowing, engaging in scientific research, and volunteering at facilities like clinics and nursing homes. These activities may have been mentioned in the application, but the medical essays often give you the opportunity to expand on your involvement with such activities.

Diligence

A third medical essay topic is one that asks for your interest in the particular program that you are applying to. Medical schools are like colleges in that they want to make sure that you have done your research and are applying to the best programs for your needs. Different medical schools have different focuses, and the burden is on you to convince the medical admissions committee that you are not just applying to every program you can find but rather are applying only to the most appropriate early admissions programs. Each medical school may also have a different focus on how teaching is done. You should match your learning style with a particular medical school.

Examine the different early acceptance programs to see which might be the most appropriate for your interests. Not all programs have a particular focus, but if you are considering an application to one that does have a focus, you want to make sure that your essay reflects your interest in that area.

Maturity

The fourth category of general medical essay is a question that tries to gauge your level of maturity. Medical schools recognize that it takes a high level of maturity to be successful in medical school. It requires even more maturity for students who wish to be successful in an EAMP. To show maturity in your essays, keep the focus on your beliefs and your actions, not on you. Communicate your answer to the question posed by being factual in discussing what you have done.

Now that you know the general topics of medical essays, let's look at some of the actual questions used by early admissions medical programs, either currently or in the past. Northwestern University's Honors Program in Medical Education (HPME) in the past asked three questions on their application.

1. *Explain the factors that are driving you toward a career in medicine.*

   This first question is the classic "why medicine" essay that virtually all of the early acceptance programs ask. While this is probably the most important essay question for you to answer, you can use the same essay at most of the programs.

2. *If you were not attending a school next year and had the freedom to dedicate the year to anything you wanted to do, what would it be?*

   Northwestern's purpose for this question is to both measure your level of maturity and to see what kind of person you are at heart. As with all of these questions, there are no right or wrong answers. What is important is to read each question carefully and answer the question asked. Your answer to a question like this does not need to be that you would spend the year doing scientific research. Tell them what your true passion is and how that passion drives you. If that passion is research, fine. But, if it involves helping those less fortunate, that is fine also.

3. *How did you deal with a situation where you didn't achieve the outcome you desired?*

   This is a simple maturity question. They are looking not only for an answer to the question but also for something that you hopefully learned from the experience.

Here is the question from Virginia Commonwealth University.

> *Comment on your motivation for, and interest in, medicine.*
> This is the "why medicine" essay. Although the question is phrased differently than Northwestern's first question, they are looking for the same information.

Union College and their program with Albany Medical College ask two questions. The first is as follows:

> *Albany Medical College seeks uniquely qualified students for the Leadership in Medicine Program. This special program focuses on three key areas that today's physicians must be prepared to address: the economic and financial problems facing medicine, including health policy and health management; the increasing complexity of biomedical ethics; and the need to maintain a global perspective. This intense program prepares physicians to provide excellent health care delivery and to take a leadership role in the rapid transformation occurring in health care management, especially in the areas of medical practice administration, organizational structures, information technology, and comprehensive medical insurance coverage.*
>
> *The Leadership in Medicine Program educates future physicians not only in the basic and clinical sciences, but also in the business/management/policy side of medicine. Please state why you are applying to this program and what uniquely qualifies you for the special focus of this program.*

This question is somewhat unusual in that it doesn't ask for the basic "why medicine" essay. Instead, it focuses on why the student would be a good applicant for their program and the specific focus that this program has. To answer this question you need to examine carefully the focus of the program as described in the preamble to the question. It may also be helpful to examine the web pages associated with the program to see if there is a further explanation of the program's focus.

The second question from the Union–Albany program is:

Describe yourself (other than scholastic achievements). (1000 character limit)

This is a generic question that allows you to enhance your application by focusing on those aspects of your life that make you a strong candidate for an early acceptance program and that have not been previously discussed in your application. Typically this may include some of the volunteer activities you have been involved with although it may also involve a discussion of your personal beliefs.

Siena College also has an EAMP with Albany Medical College. Unlike the program that Union has with Albany Medical College, the Siena College program places emphasis on humanities, ethics, and social service.

Siena's supplemental question reflects this different philosophical approach.

Describe a personal service experience in your high school or community, what you have gained from this experience, and how it reflects the unique values of the Siena College/ Albany Medical College Program.

This question has multiple parts, and you must make sure that you answer all parts of the question. You also need to do your research to make sure you understand what the unique values are of the Siena–Albany program. Typically, you should be able to find information of this type on the colleges' websites.

Here are some examples of questions from other EAMPs. The University of Rochester program has two questions.

1. *Your freshman year in college hasn't started yet, but you're applying for early acceptance to a graduate degree program. Please comment on why you feel you will be ready in a few years for the challenges of your chosen graduate program.* (limit 300)

2. *Please explore the distinct educational philosophy, area of study, or research project of a faculty member teaching in the graduate program to which you are applying. Tell us why you would enjoy working with this person. Rather than contacting a faculty member, please research the variety of print and online resources available.*

Rice University's program has three questions for applicants.

1. *What aspirations, experiences, or relationships have motivated you to study in the eight-year Rice–Baylor Medical Scholars Program?*
2. *Outside of academics, what do you enjoy doing most?*
3. *Describe the most difficult adversity you have faced, and describe how you dealt with it.*

Penn State University has two different questions for applicants.

1. *Write a personal statement indicating why you want to be a physician, why you want an accelerated program and why you've selected this Penn State / Jefferson program.* Please answer this question in 500 words or less.
2. *Describe what you think your strongest qualities are, as well as weaknesses that you would like to improve upon.*

The University of Miami asks one question.

Give a personal history of yourself, your reasons for wanting to study in your chosen field, and why you are interested in the Dual-Degree Honors Program at the University of Miami. (must be 2 pages)

Drexel University asks the following question:

Tell the Admissions Committee why you are applying to the joint program(s) with Drexel University College of Medicine. Be sure to explain why you want to be a physi-

cian and more specifically why you want to obtain your medical education at Drexel University College of Medicine. If you are applying to any of our accelerated joint programs (those with only 3 years of college), be sure to explain why you are pursuing that particular option.

The University of Connecticut asks five questions on their application.

1. *Please briefly share the influences on your decision to pursue this field of medicine.*
2. *Please describe your interests, activities, hobbies, etc. outside the area of health sciences.*
3. *Please list your work experiences paid or volunteer while in high school.*
4. *Why are you applying for the combined medical or dental program at the University of Connecticut?*
5. *Fast forward four years. Please describe what you will be like when you are a University of Connecticut senior. What will have been distinctive about your preparation for professional school?*

Brown University's Program in Liberal Medical Education (PLME) asks:

Most high school students are unsure about eventual career choices. What experiences have you to consider medicine as your future profession? Please describe specifically why you have chosen to apply to the Program in Liberal Medical Education in pursuit of your career in medicine. Also, be sure to indicate your rationale on how the PLME is a 'good fit' for your personal academic and future professional goals.

As you can see there is great variation in the questions asked by the different early acceptance programs. Moreover, the medical schools and colleges may change the questions they ask in subsequent years. However, by having some idea of the various types of questions that might be asked, you can start work on general responses before you even decide which programs you are going to apply to. Since your answer to the essay questions can be the difference between an invitation to interview and no interview, taking the additional time to work on essays may make the difference.

Chapter 5

The Medical School Interview

Congratulations! Based on your grades, test scores, activities, and essays, you have been accepted into the undergraduate college you applied to. Upon acceptance, your file is sent to the medical school admissions committee for their review. After the medical school admissions committee has reviewed all of the files, they decide which students to ask for an interview. Only those students who are asked to interview continue to be considered for acceptance into the early acceptance program.

The medical school will contact you directly to arrange a time for an interview. Some medical schools give you several dates to choose from for your interview while other programs give you a specific date for your interview and it is up to you to be there on that date. You should be aware that unlike most college interviews, medical school interviews are always conducted at the campus of the medical college. This means that if you are asked to interview for a particular program, you need to travel to that campus for your interview. It can be expensive to travel to a campus that is far from where you live, particularly if you have multiple interviews. If money is an issue, when deciding where to apply, you should carefully consider if you can afford to attend an interview on a campus far from where you live.

While getting an interview is great news, not all students given an interview will be accepted into a program. In fact, in most programs, far fewer than half of the students interviewed are accepted into the program. In this chapter we are going to look at what you can do to have a great medical school interview and improve your chances of acceptance into an early acceptance program.

Before we discuss what happens during a medical school interview, it is important that you understand what the medical school interviewers look for in a successful candidate. The primary characteristics of a successful candidate are a passion to become a physician, a high level of maturity, and interpersonal skills that allow you to become a compassionate physician. What does that mean?

The interviewers are trying to learn what you are like as a person, how you think, what your values are, and how you handle pressure. What they are evaluating with these interviews is your maturity level. Medical schools want to make sure that you are mature enough to handle the rigors of medical school as well as the rigors of being a practicing physician.

Interviewers are also looking to see how well you communicate with others. The ability to communicate with patients and other doctors is critical to be a successful physician, and your ability to speak is tested directly with the interview. Can you speak clearly and articulately? Can you answer questions in such a way that a patient will understand you?

We will look at some of the specific questions you might be asked during a medical school interview later in this chapter; but first, let's look at the basics of preparing for the medical school interview.

How to Be Successful at a Medical School Interview

There are a number of very basic things that you need to do to make sure that you have a successful medical school interview. Here is a list of things you need to do before your interview:

1. *Confirm where you need to be to begin the interview and get there early.* You do not want to be late to your

interview because you didn't know where you were going. There is no worse way to start an interview than by being late. Plan to arrive at least fifteen minutes before your scheduled interview. Also make sure that you have the proper directions to get to where you are going. Ideally, drive to the interview site the day before the interview to know exactly where you are going.

2. *Prepare for the interview by considering questions you might be asked and your answers to them, as well as questions you wish to have answered.* It is best to practice these questions and answers aloud with someone you trust to give honest feedback. Later in this chapter we will give you a list of questions that are typically asked in medical school interviews as well as a list of questions that you might consider asking of the people you speak with.

3. *Review your application and in particular all of your activities.* It is common for interviewers to ask a number of detailed questions about your activities, so you want to make sure that they are fresh in your mind. Be prepared to answer questions about not just what you did, but why you participated in that particular activity and what you learned from your participation.

4. *Learn as much as you can about the medical school you are applying to.* Medical schools, like colleges, may have different teaching styles and different personalities. Is there an emphasis on family practice or is it more of a research based medical facility? What options are there for foreign study during your time in medical school? Medical schools want to know that you are will be a serious student, committed to their institution; one way to prove this is to have done diligent research about why you are interested in that medical school in particular. Specific examples are always helpful.

5. *Dress appropriately and conservatively.* Suit and tie are always appropriate for men. Women can wear a pants suit or a skirt with a blazer. If you have piercings anywhere other than your ears, right before your interview would be a good time to remove the piercings. If you have tattoos, try to cover them up as much as possible. It is fine to show your individual spirit but piercings and tattoos are not the way to do it for medical school interviews.

6. *Turn off your cell phone before going into the interview.* This is just common courtesy. There should be nothing more important to you at this time than the interview.

7. *Bring multiple copies of your activities résumé with you.* Most interviewers have a copy of your application or activities résumé available to them, but it is always a good idea to bring a copy of your activities résumé in case the interviewer is not fully prepared.

8. *Have a firm handshake when greeting people, but not too firm.* You want to be self-assured, but you don't want to crush their hand. If need be, try practicing with multiple friends and family members beforehand.

9. *Look people in the eyes while talking with them.* This is the sign of someone who is self-confident and also indicates that you are interested in what is being said by the person you are interviewing with.

10. *Smile and be positive.* Yes, you are nervous. Yes, these programs are incredibly competitive. But during the interview you need to get past those feelings and present yourself as the strong, confident candidate that you are. If you were not a strong candidate, you wouldn't be having the interview.

11. *Listen carefully to the question asked and respond directly to that question.* When people are nervous they don't always listen to the question being asked

or they hear the first part of the question and assume they know how the question will end. Don't fall into this trap. By carefully listening to the entire question before formulating your response you will be sure to answer the question that was asked of you.

If you need a second to collect your thoughts before answering, take a deep breath and answer when you are ready. You should also be aware of how fast you are talking. When someone is nervous it is very common that they talk too fast. Slow it down so that you are having a conversation, not rushing through.

12. *Don't ramble in your answers; keep answers fairly short but responsive.* Giving a long, rambling response to a question generally indicates that you either don't have a succinct logical response or that you are nervous. Preparation is key. Make sure you are adequately prepared to answer most questions you might be asked.

13. *Don't be conceited; be self-assured but humble about your accomplishments.* No one likes someone who comes across as self-centered. At the same time, you should be confident and ready to talk about all of the strengths you have and why you would make a good candidate for the program. It can be a fine line to walk between conceited and self-assured. Practice answering questions, with someone who knows you well asking typical questions. Ask them to evaluate how you might appear to a stranger.

14. *Make sure that you come across as sincere.* Medical schools are looking for bright, mature students who can handle the work but will also be caring, compassionate physicians. Do not try to fake who you are during the interview. If you try to be someone you are not, the interviewer will most likely recognize this and will not treat you as a serious candidate.

What Will Happen during a Medical School Interview?

There is no one formula for the medical school interview process, but most interviews follow a standard pattern. You will most likely have a number of interviews during your time on campus. The interviews may just involve you and one interviewer. You may also have several interviewers asking you questions at the same time. Some programs do group interviews, where a number of prospective applicants are interviewed at the same time.

Most programs arrange for you to interview with a physician who teaches at the medical school. It is also common to interview with students who are currently in the program. The day of your interviews you will be given a tour of the medical school and often a hospital associated with the school. A lunch with students currently in the program is common. Despite the more informal nature of the tour and the lunch, you must keep in mind that these elements are also part of the interview process. Admissions offices commonly ask tour guides or students you had lunch with for their feedback on you as a student in their program. The process of going through multiple interviews and the tour generally takes most of the day, so you should not plan on doing anything other than the interviews on the day they have been arranged.

The Interviewers

We mentioned that you may be interviewed by a physician who teaches in the program or by past or current students of the program. Try to find out before the day of the interview who you will be interviewing with. If you are able to do so, do some research to learn what you can about your interviewer's professional life. Where did they go to college and medical school? What is their medical specialty? Have they been involved in research and published papers? Knowing something about your interviewer helps you feel at ease and gives you topics to discuss with your interviewer. It also shows that you are motivated enough to do the research about your interviewer.

Most of the people interviewing you for these combined degree programs will be friendly and trying to put you at ease. They really do want to get to know you to see if you are a good candidate for their program. However, different people use different interviewing techniques. Some questioners may get aggressive during the interview to see how you handle pressure. Don't become upset if this happens to you. Keep your cool, and don't get defensive. Answer the questions in a calm and respectful manner. Medicine can be stressful, and if you are able to remain calm during the interview, it shows that you can handle the stress without breaking down.

Questions You Should Be Prepared to Answer

There are literally thousands of questions that you might be asked during the medical school interview process. But don't panic. Most of the questions fall into a particular category of question. Knowing the major types of questions will help you answer any question you are asked. The first four categories of questions revolve around you and your résumé. Categories five through eight focus more on why you wish to be a doctor. Finally, the interview will end with open-ended questions so you can learn more about the medical school where you are interviewing.

While many interviewers follow this general order in asking questions, there are no rules that they need to follow in asking you questions. Some interviewers jump right into the question of why you wish to become a doctor. Don't worry about the order in which you might be asked questions. Rather, make sure that you understand the categories of questions and that you are prepared to answer questions related to each of the categories, regardless of the order of the questions.

1. General questions about you and your activities

Most questioners will start the interview asking general questions about you and the activities you have participated in during high school. You should carefully review your résumé before attending the interview. Here are typical questions that may be asked about you and your activities:

> What can you tell me about yourself?
> What do you do for enjoyment?
> What are the last three books you read?
> What magazines do you read?
> What is your greatest strength or weakness?
> How do you spend your free time?

2. Questions about your research experiences

Most students who are competitive for BS/MD programs have some type of research they have participated in before applying to these programs. You may be asked questions about the research you did. Typically, you need to discuss the specifics of what you did during the research, what the purpose of the research was, and the findings of the research. The most important point is that you must be prepared to show you fully understand the nature of your research project. These questions are meant to confirm that you have a real interest in the research you engaged in and did not just do it to enhance your résumé. You may also be asked to describe a problem you faced when you were conducting the research and to tell how you worked to overcome or solve it.

3. Questions about your doctor shadowing experiences

Your application should have detailed your involvement with shadowing one or more physicians while they were working. You may be asked questions about this experience including what you did during the shadowing, what medical problems you were exposed to, and whether the doctors you worked with influenced your outlook on a career in medicine?

The types of medical problems you observed are not as important as the experience you had following the doctor.

4. Questions about your volunteer activities

Most interviewers will ask you questions about your volunteer activities. These questions are important because your answers tell the interviewer something about your compassion. Compassion is a major factor that BS/MD programs are looking for in applicants. They want students who are concerned about others, and not just about themselves and how much money they can make as a physician. Your answers to these questions allow you to expand on what is hopefully your sincere desire to work for the betterment of others.

You may discuss not only what you did with your volunteer work but also what your motivation was in volunteering at this facility. You might discuss how you felt after volunteering.

Most students have some of their volunteer activities in health-related fields, so you can also use these questions to reinforce your understanding of the health care field and your commitment to becoming a physician.

If you do not have a long-term (more than one year) commitment to a particular volunteer program, and you have a good reason for this, now is your chance to explain why you don't have the long-term involvement.

5. *Questions about why you want to be a doctor*

Why do you want to be a doctor?

No matter which program you are interviewing for or who is asking the questions, this question, or some variation of it, is the central part of your interview. It is critical that you have a good answer to this question prepared before your interview. Why is this question so important?

This question allows the interviewer to assess your motivation to become a physician. Are you passionate about becoming a physician? Have you really thought about what it means to be a doctor? Do you understand how rigorous the training is and what an effect being a doctor has on your lifestyle? Are you ready, as a high school senior, to commit yourself to a career in medicine?

A similar question that often is asked during an interview is, When did you first decide on medicine as a profession? Most students applying to BS/MD programs have wanted to become a doctor for many years. What is important in answering this question is that you communicate that you have given a great deal of thought to your chosen profession.

What will you do if you are not admitted to the BS/MD program is another common question that may be asked of you. The best answer is that you will continue to work toward your goal of becoming a doctor by taking the traditional route to medical school. You want to communicate that your ultimate goal is to become a doctor. While you would prefer the BS/MD route, you are not willing to give up your dream just because you might not get into one of these programs. That shows dedication and maturity.

A related question is, What would you do if you are not accepted into medical school at all? In asking this question, the interviewer is seeing whether you are focused on science-related fields even if medical school is not possible. Your answer does not necessarily need to be employment in a science-related field if your focus is on other fields where you may be able to help people. Remember, passion and compassion.

Here are some other questions that you might be asked that relate to the category of your interest in medicine:

> What type of doctor do you want to be and why?
> Are you more interested in a clinical practice or research? Why do you have an interest in that type of medicine?
> What strengths or qualities do you have that will help make you a good physician?
> What qualities should a good physician have?
> What do you think you will like about medicine? What will you dislike?
> What challenges do you think you will face during your medical career?

You want to establish your passion and compassion. But, it is not enough to use these buzz words. Use stories and examples from your life to show that you have the passion and compassion that will make you a great physician. You do not need to ever even say the words passion and compassion if the stories you tell establish that this is who you are. Think about who you are and how your life exhibits these two traits before the interview. Then let your story do the convincing.

6. Questions about why you want to do a combined BS/MD program rather than the traditional route.

We have already discussed how competitive these programs are and how much of the admissions process revolves around your proving your serious interest in a career in medicine. However, the vast majority of students, including those who have had a dream for years of becoming a doctor, still go the traditional route to become a doctor. Why do you think a combined BS/MD program is preferable for you?

There are many reasons you may think such a program is in your best interest. You may like the accelerated program because it allows you to reach your goal of becoming a physician sooner. Keep in mind, most of these BS/MD programs are not accelerated, and it takes you the traditional eight years to complete college and medical school. If you are applying to an accelerated program, then this answer is fine, but if you are applying to one of the eight-year programs, this type of answer shows that you don't know enough about the program you have applied to.

The most common answer to this type of question is that an early acceptance into medical school takes much of the pressure off you during your college years. You don't have to worry about grades as much as the traditional students, who are competing with each other to see who can get the best grades. As previously mentioned, the minimum grade point averages required of most programs is around a 3.5 GPA. Students who are qualified for these programs rarely have a problem receiving an average 3.5 GPA.

In a BS/MD program, you also have more flexibility to take classes that are of interest to you and that are not just focused on the sciences. Most of the eight-year BS/MD programs have no problem with their students taking classes outside the sciences, and in fact many encourage academic exploration. They understand that a well-rounded student will often have an easier time communicating with patients than one who spent all four years of college in a science lab.

Students in these programs often have additional benefits such as early experiences at the medical school or enhanced research experiences. Brown University's Program in Liberal Medical Education (PLME), for instance, has the Medicine in Action program, where undergraduates and medical students can "explore a variety of clinical settings, observe physician/patient relationships firsthand, go on rounds with the medical team, and get to know individual medical school faculty and alumni more closely. Medical students are offered the opportunity to hone their career choices by seeking mentors in their area of interest." Opportunities like this can greatly enhance a student's medical education.

Finally, some programs do not require their students to take the MCAT before medical school, or the required score on the MCAT is eased for those in the program. This alleviates much of the stress related to taking this high stakes test that those not in the program will need to experience.

7. Questions about why you are interested in this particular program

In Chapter 3, we discussed the different types of programs and the unique nature of each program. The questions in this category ensure you have applied to the right program for you. There can be overlap between the answers to these types of questions and those that ask why you want a BS/MD program. For instance, as we just discussed, the PLME program at Brown provides certain additional program options for its students. You should investigate what additional educational opportunities each program makes available so that you are prepared to discuss your interest in that type of program.

Some BS/MD programs also have a particular focus, and if you have an interest in the focus of that program, now is the time to discuss your interest. For instance, Union College and Albany Medical College have a joint BS/MD program known as the Leadership in Medicine Program. This program emphasizes undergraduate training in the sciences as well as humanities and health care management. This would be a good program for those students interested in medicine as well as health care management.

Albany Medical College also has a program with Rensselaer Polytechnic Institute called the Physician Scientist Program. This seven-year program has a goal to "prepare physicians who will advance the practice of medicine through their clinical skills combined with their understanding and ability to carry out health care research."

Although each of these programs uses Albany Medical College, it should be clear that a single student would not likely be a good choice for both programs. Choosing the right programs to apply to becomes particularly important when this question is asked of you. And if you think you can just fake an answer, the interviewer is looking at your entire résumé to see if it is consistent with the focus of this program. If you claim to have an interest in the Rensselaer program, your résumé should contain several examples of your interest in scientific research.

Here are some examples of questions that you might be asked, to determine whether this is the right program for you.

Why are you applying to this BS/MD program and in particular this medical school?
Where else have you applied?
What's your first choice and why?
What qualities do you have that other applicants don't?
How are you a good match for our medical school?
What makes you unique?
What criteria are you using to evaluate potential medical schools?

8. Questions about current medical issues and ethics

Most interviewers will ask you at least one question related to a current topic in medical ethics. Common topics include embryonic stem cell research, medical malpractice, socialized medicine, genetic engineering, abortion, physician assisted suicide, euthanasia and other end of life issues.

There are several purposes for these questions. First, the interviewer is seeing whether you have knowledge of current medical issues. Most students who have a passion for medi-

Final Thoughts

Preparation is the key to a successful interview. If you have seriously read through this chapter, have understood the categories of questions you might be asked, and have thought about answers to each of the categories, you should be well prepared for your interview. During the interview keep two key words in the back of your head; passion and compassion. In answering each question consider how your answer demonstrates your passion for becoming a physician and the compassion that will make you a great physician.

And don't forget to thank the interviewer.

Chapter 6

Paying for Early Medical Programs

Four years of college followed by four years of medical school is very expensive. Even if you are looking at one of the programs that is six or seven years long, there is a tremendous cost associated with medical school. If you are fortunate to come from a family that can easily afford this, then skip ahead to Chapter 7. Otherwise, let's talk about paying for college and medical school.

Paying for College

There are three types of financial aid for college: grants or scholarships, loans, and work-study.

GRANTS AND SCHOLARSHIPS are free money that you do not need to pay back. Most grants and scholarships come from the federal and state government or from the individual college.

LOANS need to be paid back after college. There are many loan programs available from the federal and state governments. Most of these loans have fairly low interest rates. There are also private loans available, although these generally have a higher interest rate and are much less desirable.

WORK-STUDY is a job offered on the campus of the college.

You also need to understand the difference between need-based aid and merit-based aid.

NEED-BASED AID is given by all colleges to students who have need. Anyone who can't pay the full cost of the college has need. A form called the Free Application for Federal Student Aid (FAFSA) determines the amount of need for federal grants and scholarships. The FAFSA form is filled out after January 1 of the year you will first attend college. Many highly selective colleges also require a form known as the CSS Profile form.

The FAFSA and Profile forms ask questions about your and your parents' income, using information that you gave on your tax returns. These forms also ask questions about the amount of money you have in savings or investments. The Profile form is more detailed than the FAFSA form. The government uses the FAFSA form to determine how much your family can pay for college. This is your expected family contribution or your EFC. Your EFC is the same regardless of the cost of the college. Similarly, the individual colleges who use the Profile use that form to determine what your family can pay for college.

Your need is the cost of the college you are looking at minus your EFC. For example, if you are looking at a college that costs $20,000 a year and your EFC is $5,000, your need at that college is $15,000. If you are looking at a college that costs $50,000 a year your EFC is still $5,000, your need at this college is $45,000.

MERIT-BASED AID includes scholarships typically for students who have good grades or have some other special ability, such as athletic or musical talent. Most highly selective colleges offer little or no merit-based aid.

Finally, in looking at colleges you should ignore the cost of the college. Yes, you read that right. Ignore the stated cost of the college when you are first deciding which colleges to investigate further. You will see why later in this chapter.

So now you know the basics. However, each college handles financial aid a bit differently. You need to understand how the particular colleges you are looking at handle financial aid. To know that, you need to ask some questions.

Question 1: What percent of my need do you meet?

Remember that EFC, or expected family contribution that the FAFSA determined? Some colleges will meet one hundred percent of your need. Need again is defined as the cost of the college minus your EFC. So what does it mean if a college says they will meet one hundred percent of your need? It means that once the FAFSA or Profile form has determined how much you can pay for college, the college will pay the rest of the bill.

Colleges typically meet the need you have using a combination of grants, loans, and work-study. Most colleges award work-study and loans first, and if there is a need after that, the remaining need is supplied by grants. The colleges typically have a standard loan and work-study amount that they award, and you should ask about what these numbers are when investigating the college.

Let's see an example of a financial aid award from a college that provides one hundred percent of need, with a student who has an EFC of $5,000.

Total cost of college	$50,000
Family's expected contribution	5,000
Need	45,000
Financial aid award	
Work-study	2,000
Loans	4,000
Grants	39,000

At a college that meets one hundred percent of your need you pay $5,000.

But what happens if the college doesn't meet 100% of need?

Many less selective colleges don't pay the total amount of need that their students have under their need-based aid programs. Keep in mind that when we talk about a less selective college, we are talking about a regular application to a college, not one for a college's BS/MD program. Many undergraduate colleges that have BS/MD programs are not very selective for their regular admissions. In most colleges, financial aid is handled the same for its regular applicants and those applying to the BS/MD program.

Let's use the example of our imaginary college from above, only this time assume that the school only provides eighty percent of need.

Total cost of college	$50,000
Family's expected contribution	5,000
Need	45,000

This college only provides eighty percent of the $45,000 need or $36,000. Thus, your out-of-pocket expenses are the $5,000 EFC plus an additional $9,000, for a total cost of $14,000.

This example makes it easy to see why a school that meets one hundred percent of need is often a better financial aid deal than a school that doesn't meet all of the family's need.

Many of the most expensive private colleges meet one hundred percent of the student's need, while cheaper public colleges usually meet less than one hundred percent of the need. This means that for many students it can be cheaper to go to an expensive private college than to attend a cheaper state school. Until you know what percent of need the college meets, don't eliminate a college from consideration just because it is expensive.

Question 2: Do you have merit-based aid?

Many colleges that don't meet one hundred percent of a student's need do offer scholarships for some students. If you are near the top of the application pool for a less selective college, you may get some money if you qualify for merit-based aid. At most colleges that offer a BS/MD program, the applicants to these programs are among the most talented students at that college, and they will often be considered for merit-based aid. Here are some questions you should ask if the college provides merit aid.

> How many merit awards are available?
> What is the value of the merit awards available?
> What are the qualifications to receive one of these merit awards?

This works even for families that don't qualify for need-based aid at all. If you can qualify for a merit-based award, you won't need to pay the full stated cost of the college.

Question 3: How is financial aid determined after the first year?

Some colleges have a policy of providing good financial aid for the first year and then substantially reducing the grant aid in the following years while increasing the loans. You should ask the college in which you are interested how they determine financial aid after the first year and what the average loan is after the first year. While it is typical that the amount of loans will increase each year, if the increase is substantial, you want to take that into consideration.

Question 4: What is the average loan amount at graduation of those students who have loans?

This question will give you the best indication of the amount of loans that this college requires compared to other colleges in which you may be interested. Although most students will have some loans when they graduate, you don't want this amount to be any more than necessary. This is particularly true for students who plan to go to medical school, as loans are the primary form of financial aid for medical school.

Question 5: What is your policy regarding outside scholarships?

Most colleges subtract money earned in outside scholarships from your financial aid package. Some colleges reduce the loan burden by the amount of the scholarship, but other colleges reduce your grant money. If the college reduces the amount of loans you have to take out, that is a benefit to you. There is no benefit to you if the college reduces the grant aid.

Question 6: What is your packaging policy?

Most colleges give a financial aid package that includes grant money, loans, and work-study. But each college combines this money differently. Specifically you want to know:

What percentage of an aid package from your college is grant vs. self-help (that is, loans and work-study)?

The greater amount of grants relative to loans and work-study, the better for the student.

Paying for Medical School

At most medical schools, the primary way of paying for your education is through loans. Most loans are available from the federal government, although many states also have loans available. To qualify for these loans, you need to complete the FAFSA. In calculating your qualification for loans, most colleges do not expect any contribution from your family.

At some of the most selective schools, there are grants available to help pay for medical school. Such grants are available to those families with lower income levels. However, medical schools that have grant money available generally consider the income and assets of the student's parents and not just the student.

At a few of the medical schools that have grant money available, families with lower income levels may not have to contribute as much to the education as would otherwise be the case. For example, Harvard Medical School expects no family contribution from parents with income less than $120,000. However, this sort of financial aid is the exception when dealing with paying for medical school.

The majority of students paying for medical school will do so using loans entirely. Although this may seem like a huge burden, and it is, the expectation is that once medical students graduate and start making money, they will have enough resources to pay off the loans.

Chapter 7

Other Issues
Related to BS/MD Admissions

Acceptance of International Students into Early Acceptance Programs

Many international students are interested in admissions to BS/MD programs, but there are limited options for these students. Most of the BS/MD programs only accept students who are United States citizens or permanent residents of the United States.

There are a few BS/MD programs that consider international students, including the program at Northwestern University and the program at Brown University. International applicants should keep in mind that as competitive as these programs are for U.S. citizens, they are even more competitive for international students. International students who are interested in applying to the few programs available to them must also have other plans for college made, in case they are not accepted into one of the BS/MD programs.

The appendix lists information on each of the BS/MD programs in the U.S., including a note for those that will consider international students.

Acceptance of Transfer Students

Most BS/MD programs only accept applications from students who are incoming freshmen. Transfer applications are specifically not accepted. A limited number of BS/MD programs accept transfer students. Those that do accept transfer students typically do so only after the first year of undergraduate education. Those programs that consider transfer applications are noted in the appendix.

How Many Programs Should You Apply To?

There is no magic number of BS/MD programs that a student should apply to. Contrary to popular belief, more is not necessarily better. While the typical program may only accept one out of twenty students who apply, that does not mean that if you apply to twenty programs you will get into at least one.

Just like choosing a regular college, you want to look at what you want from a college, or BS/MD program, and then find programs that fit your needs. Remember Chapter 3, where we discussed what to look for in a program. That is your starting point. The typical student with whom we work applies to eight to ten BS/MD programs. You should also consider applying to at least six to ten regular colleges that have a strong history of science education and medical school placement. While twelve to fifteen colleges is a huge number of applications, and many more than we recommend for students looking at traditional colleges, it is a good number to consider based on our experiences with students applying to BS/MD programs.

Applying to Traditional College Programs

One final, but very important, note. Because the BS/MD programs are so competitive, every student applying to such a program must also apply to several traditional four-year colleges in case they are not accepted into a BS/MD program. The regular college list should include some colleges in which you are fairly sure you will gain acceptance. These are colleges that many people refer to as safety schools. It should not be a problem to find some good colleges for this purpose, since students who are competitive for BS/MD programs are such strong students.

The focus on the search for traditional colleges should be on colleges that have historically done well in educating their students and preparing them for medical school. This list often includes smaller liberal arts colleges, which are among the most successful colleges in medical school placement.

Some students will want to apply only to the BS/MD programs, with the thought that they are likely to be admitted to most of the undergraduate programs even if they are not admitted to the BS/MD program. They figure that they can always just attend the undergraduate college of the BS/MD program as their college option. This is generally not a good idea. Although some of the undergraduate programs are by themselves good schools to prepare for medical school, many of the undergraduate programs associated with the BS/MD programs are not as academically strong. Students should consider the regular college list as completely separate from the BS/MD list. This way, they are more likely to have regular colleges on their list that do a good job of preparation for medical school rather than colleges that might do an okay job of preparation for medical school.

BS/MD Programs by State

The information provided in the appendix is believed to be accurate as of the date of the publication of this book. However, BS/MD programs are constantly being started while others are being discontinued. Also, the information regarding minimal grades and test scores as well as the dates applications are required are subject to change at any time. If you find a program in which you have an interest, go to the website of that program to verify information. For updated information you can check our website: www.collegeadmissionspartners.com/bsmd-admissions/.

There is some inconsistency in the way GPA and test scores are reported. Some schools list only their minimum requirements. Some list the averages for *accepted* students. Others list the averages for *enrolled* students. These two averages are not interchangeable. Typically the averages for accepted students are higher than those for enrolled students.

NOTE ON FINANCIAL AID AND COSTS Information about financial aid is listed only if there is a special program available for students admitted to the program. The listed costs are generally for tuition and fees only, although some programs include room and board costs as part of a total package. For more detail about the cost of each program, see the website of each school.

The information provided regarding each school varies in depth depending on the information made available to us by the different programs. Some are more transparent than others and may have more information. We have updated admissions information where available.

NOTE ON THE ARRANGEMENT OF THIS APPENDIX Programs are alphabetical by the state where the medical school is, and then alphabetical by associated undergraduate college.

COLLEGE

University of Alabama Birmingham

MEDICAL SCHOOL

University of Alabama School of Medicine

ADDRESS

UAB Honors Academy, HUC 531
University of Alabama at Birmingham
1530 Third Avenue South
Birmingham, Alabama 35294-1150
800-421-8743; 205-934-8221
www.uab.edu/emsap/
chooseuab@uab.edu

NAME OF PROGRAM

Early Medical School Acceptance Program (EMSAP)

LENGTH OF PROGRAM

8 years

APPLICATION DEADLINE

You must be admitted to the university and complete the honors application by December 1. The Early Medical School Acceptance Program application is due December 15.

INFORMATION ABOUT THE PROGRAM

Students may major in any of the fifty-three majors offered by the college. Regardless of your major, the program will also make sure you fulfill the prerequisites for the medical school.

Special seminars are offered to students in the program, and a student is required to take at least two seminars before medical school. The seminars focus on themes such as medical ethics, reproductive biology, and the history of medicine. Quarterly meetings provide an opportunity to discuss health care issues and to talk with alumni of the program.

Numerous clinical experiences are made available, including research, patient care, doctor shadowing, and work in laboratories. Volunteer service at a local health care facility is required as part of the program.

There is some attrition with this program. About fifteen percent of the students admitted to the program fail out. In addition, about fifty percent are on probation at some time during the undergraduate years.

This program does allow students to apply out to other medical schools without losing their guaranteed spot in the medical school.

UAB changed their interview technique in 2015 to include a multiple mini-interview model where students will be presented with problem solving scenarios at a variety of stations in addition to a traditional long-form interview.

TRANSFER STUDENTS CONSIDERED

No

CITIZENSHIP REQUIREMENTS

U.S. citizen or permanent resident visa

MINIMUM REQUIRED FACTORS IN SELECTION

CLASSES

Four years of English and math, one year of chemistry or physics, and one year of biology

GPA

3.5 unweighted. Average accepted GPA 4.49 weighted.

SAT

1,340 critical reading and math. Average accepted 1,450.

ACT

30. Average accepted ACT 33.7.

ACCEPTANCES

EMSAP typically recieves over 200 applications. They interview up to 30 students for 10 spots; traditionally about half are Alabama residents.

FACTORS REQUIRED TO CONTINUE IN PROGRAM

3.5 or higher GPA in natural science and math courses; overall GPA of 3.6 or higher

MCAT REQUIRED

Yes; minimum score of 28

FINANCIAL AID

No special financial aid for students in the program; most students qualify for merit-based scholarships based on GPA and test scores.

COST

	Resident Tuition and Fees ($)	Non Resident Tuition and Fees ($)
Undergraduate	9,596	21,956
Medical school	29,048	64,514

COLLEGE
University of South Alabama

MEDICAL SCHOOL
University of South Alabama College of Medicine

ADDRESS
University of South Alabama
Meisler Hall, Room 2500
Mobile, Alabama 36688-0022
251-460-6141
www.southalabama.edu/departments/admissions
/comearlyacceptance.html
recruitment@southalabama.edu

NAME OF PROGRAM
College of Medicine Early Acceptance Program (EAP)

LENGTH OF PROGRAM
8 years

APPLICATION DEADLINE
January 15.

INFORMATION ABOUT THE PROGRAM
Students in the program are required to participate for four semesters in a course entitled Career Planning: Clinical Observation. Students are given the opportunity to participate in a two-week summer clerkship in a clinical setting. The purpose of the clerkship is to provide a positive clinical experience with a practicing physician.

Students in the program will be reviewed at the end of each year by the Health Pre-Professions Advisor and a committee of admissions from the medical school to confirm that academic requirements have been met.

TRANSFER STUDENTS CONSIDERED
No

CITIZENSHIP REQUIREMENTS
U.S. citizen or permanent resident visa. Preference is given to residents of Alabama and certain areas of Florida and Mississippi. Non-Alabama residents must establish Alabama residency while in the undergraduate program.

MINIMUM REQUIRED FACTORS IN SELECTION

CLASSES

No specific requirement

GPA

3.5 unweighted

SAT

1,220 critical reading and math

ACT

27

ACCEPTANCES

Typically interview 40–45 students for aproximately 15 spots.

FACTORS REQUIRED TO CONTINUE IN PROGRAM

3.4 or higher GPA in natural science and math courses; overall GPA of 3.5 or higher

MCAT REQUIRED

Yes; minimum score of 28

FINANCIAL AID

There are no special financial aid funds for students in the program

COST

	Resident Tuition and Fees ($)	Non Resident Tuition and Fees ($)
Undergraduate	6,948	13,596
Medical school	27,393	54,010

COLLEGE

California Northstate University

MEDICAL SCHOOL

California Northstate University College of Medicine

ADDRESS

California Northstate University
2910 Prospect Park Drive
Rancho Cordova, California 95670
916-686-7400
http://healthsciences.cnsu.edu/programs-offered
/bs-md-combined-program/about
admissions.chs@cnsu.edu

NAME OF PROGRAM

BS-MD Combined Program

LENGTH OF PROGRAM

6 or 7 years

APPLICATION DEADLINE

December 15

INFORMATION ABOUT THE PROGRAM

This is a brand new program starting the 2016–2017 school year. Students have an option of pursuing a six-year or seven-year combined degree path.

Students will complete their two- or three-year undergraduate study in the College of Health Sciences. Students are required to participate in a minimum of one College of Medicine activity per year, which includes career exploration, community service, and lab research opportunities.

Students on the six-year track have required summer courses, while those on the seven-year track have an option for summer classes.

TRANSFER STUDENTS CONSIDERED

No

CITIZENSHIP REQUIREMENTS

U.S. citizen or permanent resident visa

MINIMUM REQUIRED FACTORS IN SELECTION

CLASSES

No specific requirement

GPA

3.75 minimum for the six-year program; 3.60 minimum for the seven-year option

SAT

1,360 math and critical reading for the six-year program; 1,290 for the seven-year option

ACT

32 minimum for the six-year program; 29 for the seven-year option

FACTORS REQUIRED TO CONTINUE IN PROGRAM

3.5 overall GPA

MCAT REQUIRED

Yes; minimum score of 510 on the new MCAT

FINANCIAL AID

No special financial aid for students in the program

COST

	Resident Tuition and Fees ($)	Non Resident Tuition and Fees ($)
Undergraduate	29,836	29,836
Medical school	55,502	55,502

COLLEGE

University of Colorado Denver

MEDICAL SCHOOL

University of Colorado School of Medicine

ADDRESS

University of Colorado Denver School of Medicine
BA/BS-MD Program
13120 East 19th Avenue, Room 5231
Mail Stop C292
Aurora, Colorado 80045
303-352-3557
www.ucdenver.edu/academics/colleges/CLAS/BachelorsPrograms
/ProgramsDegrees/BABSMD/Pages/home.aspx
babsmd@ucdenver.edu

NAME OF PROGRAM

BA/BS-MD Program

LENGTH OF PROGRAM

8 years

APPLICATION DEADLINE

October 30 for general university deadline

INFORMATION ABOUT THE PROGRAM

The program prioritizes students from under-represented minorities or from rural or financially disadvantaged backgrounds who are committed to serving the health care needs of Colorado, especially with a focus on primary care.

Students may major in any subject offered by the university. The summer before starting college students participate in a one-week bridge program. In the summer after freshman year students spend eight weeks working in hospitals or clinics in the Denver area. The summer after sophomore year students participate in a research practicum. The summer after junior year students participate in an MCAT prep course. Students are paid for their time in the summer programs. Students are required to attend monthly co-curricular seminars at the medical school.

Students first apply to the undergraduate college, and only after acceptance can they apply to the BS/MD program.

TRANSFER STUDENTS CONSIDERED

No

CITIZENSHIP REQUIREMENTS

U.S. citizen or permanent resident visa; Colorado residents only

MINIMUM REQUIRED FACTORS IN SELECTION

CLASSES

No specific requirement

GPA

3.5 and a CCHE score of 110 or better

SAT

None listed. In past years it has been 1,050.

ACT

None listed. In past years it has been 23.

ACCEPTANCES

10 students are accepted per year.

FACTORS REQUIRED TO CONTINUE IN PROGRAM

3.5 overall GPA with no grade lower than B in any medical school prerequisite course

MCAT REQUIRED

Yes; Minimum score is still being developed for new MCAT.

FINANCIAL AID

No special financial aid for students in the program, although special help is provided by the financial aid office to find additional aid and apply for available scholarships

COST

	Resident Tuition and Fees ($)	Non Resident Tuition and Fees ($)
Undergraduate	10,044	not applicable
Medical school	34,639	not applicable

COLLEGE
University of Connecticut at Storrs

MEDICAL SCHOOL
University of Connecticut School of Medicine

ADDRESS
Special Programs in Medicine and Dental Medicine
University of Connecticut
2131 Hillside Road, U-88
Storrs, Connecticut 06269-3088
860-486-3137
http://medicine.uchc.edu/prospective/babs_md/
admissions@uchc.edu

NAME OF PROGRAM
B.A./B.S. and M.D. Special Program in Medicine (SPiM)

LENGTH OF PROGRAM
8 years

APPLICATION DEADLINE
December 1

INFORMATION ABOUT THE PROGRAM
Students are allowed to complete any major offered by the university and are encouraged to explore a wide range of undergraduate courses. As undergraduates, students in the program are offered opportunities to engage in research and clinical experiences. This may include summer research at the UConn health center, clinical experience at the school of medicine, attendance at research meetings, and community service activities through the health center. During undergraduate years, students are required to engage in extra curricular community service in addition to clinical and research experiences.

TRANSFER STUDENTS CONSIDERED
No

CITIZENSHIP REQUIREMENTS
International students considered. Connecticut students given preference in admissions.

MINIMUM REQUIRED FACTORS IN SELECTION

CLASSES

No specific requirement

GPA

3.5 unweighted

SAT

1,300, 650 minimum on critical reading and 650 minimum on math

ACT

29

ACCEPTANCES

SPiM typically recieves 200–300 applications. They interview 30–40 students for approximately 15 spots. Traditionally more than 75 percent of accepted students are Connecticut residents.

FACTORS REQUIRED TO CONTINUE IN PROGRAM

3.6 GPA; participation in clinical, research, and community activities; and a favorable interview with the medical school during the senior year of college

MCAT REQUIRED

Yes; minimum score of 30 with section scores of 8 or better

FINANCIAL AID

All enrolled students considered for merit-based scholarships.

COST

	Resident Tuition and Fees ($)	Non Resident Tuition and Fees ($)
Undergraduate	12,760	32,940
Medical school	35,622	65,630

COLLEGE

George Washington University

MEDICAL SCHOOL

George Washington University School of Medicine
and Health Sciences

ADDRESS

Office of Undergraduate Admissions
The George Washington University
2121 I Street NW Suite 201
Washington, DC 20052
202-994-6040
http://undergraduate.admissions.gwu.edu/seven-year-bamd
gwadm@gwu.edu

NAME OF PROGRAM

Seven Year BA/MD Program

LENGTH OF PROGRAM

7 years

APPLICATION DEADLINE

December 1

INFORMATION ABOUT THE PROGRAM

Seminars and health care experiences are made available to students in the program. Students may arrange their program to have a period of study abroad. During the first three years of the program, a student must complete a major and meet all general curriculum requirements. A community service project is required each year. Students are supported by an undergraduate BA/MD advisor, the assistant dean of admissions at the school of medicine, and student mentors in the program. Progress through the program is reviewed annually. This program is unique, as the BA degree is awarded at the end of the three-year undergraduate experience.

A review committee meets at the end of the third year to make a final recommendation regarding admission to the medical school. This recommendation will be given if the student has met all of the requirements of the program.

TRANSFER STUDENTS CONSIDERED

No

CITIZENSHIP REQUIREMENTS

U.S. citizen or permanent resident visa; Canadian citizens also considered; some preference is given to residents of the District of Columbia, Virginia, and Maryland.

MINIMUM REQUIRED FACTORS IN SELECTION

CLASSES

No specific requirement

GPA

No specific requirement; competitive students will be in the top ten percent of their high school class.

SAT

No specific requirement; competitive scores are 2,100 and higher; SAT subject exam in one of the sciences and one in math are required

ACT

No specific requirement

ACCEPTANCES

Admitance is among the most selective, with typically around 1,000 applications for approximately 10 spots in the program.

FACTORS REQUIRED TO CONTINUE IN PROGRAM

Overall 3.6 GPA; minimum grade of B in courses required for admission to medical school; completion of a major at the college

MCAT REQUIRED

No

FINANCIAL AID

Students in the program pay a fixed undergraduate tuition rate for the first three years of the program.

COST

	Resident Tuition and Fees ($)	Non Resident Tuition and Fees ($)
Undergraduate	50,435	50,435
Medical school	55,736	55,736

COLLEGE

St. Bonaventure

MEDICAL SCHOOL

George Washington University School of Medicine and Health Sciences

ADDRESS

Director, Franciscan Health Care Professions
Biology Department, De La Roche Hall Room 219
St. Bonaventure, New York 14778
716-375-2656
www.sbu.edu/academics/schools/arts-and-sciences
/departments-majors-minors/pre-medicine
/sbu-gw-dual-admit-program-in-medicine-(m-d-)
fhcp@sbu.edu

NAME OF PROGRAM

B.S./B.A.-M.D. 4+4 Dual Admissions Program

LENGTH OF PROGRAM

8 years

APPLICATION DEADLINE

Dec. 1; last-minute applications may hurt admissions chances.

INFORMATION ABOUT THE PROGRAM

Qualified applicants are invited for an interview at St. Bonaventure in January. Students who pass this interview are invited for an interview at the George Washington Medical School in late February to early March. Acceptance decisions are made in mid to late March.

Community service and clinical experience are explicitly taken into consideration for admission to the program. At least two teacher recommendations are required, and one of them must be from a science teacher. Letters from non-teachers, such as employers, coaches, or volunteer coordinators, are encouraged.

You are required to write a personal statement outlining your interest in medicine and your particular interest in St. Bonaventure and George Washington University.

A résumé of all of your extracurricular activities is also required.

TRANSFER STUDENTS CONSIDERED

No

CITIZENSHIP REQUIREMENTS

U.S. citizen or permanent resident visa; Canadian citizens also considered

MINIMUM REQUIRED FACTORS IN SELECTION

CLASSES

No specific requirement

GPA

90 or higher, top ten percent of class

SAT

1,800; SAT subject exam in a science (biology M is preferred; chemistry is acceptable)

ACT

29

ACCEPTANCES

Typically accept 10–15 new students per year

FACTORS REQUIRED TO CONTINUE IN PROGRAM

Must be a full-time student; minimum 3.6 GPA in all science courses and overall; grade of B– or better in all courses; completion of core science and English requirements; maintaining character and comportment requirements

MCAT REQUIRED

No

FINANCIAL AID

Scholarship is available for the undergraduate years.

COST

	Resident Tuition and Fees ($)	Non Resident Tuition and Fees ($)
Undergraduate	31,389	31,389
Medical school	55,736	55,736

COLLEGE
Howard University

MEDICAL SCHOOL
Howard University College of Medicine

ADDRESS
Preprofessional Advisor
Center for Preprofessional Education
College of Arts and Sciences
Howard University
2225 Georgia Avenue NW Room 518
Washington, DC 20059-1014
202-238-2363
www.coas.howard.edu/preprofessionaleducation
/bsmd_brochure_jan2015.pdf

NAME OF PROGRAM
B.S./M.D. Accelerated Medical Education Program

LENGTH OF PROGRAM
6 years

APPLICATION DEADLINE
March 1; must already have applied and been admitted to the College of Arts and Sciences

INFORMATION ABOUT THE PROGRAM
While all students will be considered for this program, Howard University is a historically black college and has an emphasis on increasing the number of African-American physicians. Besides academics, the admissions committee considers superior writing skills, maturity, positive self-confidence, leadership skills, and volunteer efforts.

While students may be admitted to the program as high school seniors, they are reevaluated for admission to the medical program after taking the MCAT in April of the sophomore year. At that time the committee also considers whether the student has shown a high level of maturity and a strong commitment to working in an area where there is a shortage of physicians.

TRANSFER STUDENTS CONSIDERED
No

CITIZENSHIP REQUIREMENTS
U.S. citizen or permanent resident visa

MINIMUM REQUIRED FACTORS IN SELECTION

CLASSES

Two years of a foreign language, biology, chemistry, physics, algebra, geometry, and trigonometry.

GPA

3.5 minimum; average 3.7 GPA for students accepted into program

SAT

1,950; average of 2,040 for students accepted into program

ACT

26; average above 31

ACCEPTANCES

Approximately 15 new students are admitted each year.

FACTORS REQUIRED TO CONTINUE IN PROGRAM

Minimum science GPA 3.25, overall GPA 3.50

MCAT REQUIRED

Yes, minimum 24

FINANCIAL AID

No special financial aid for students in the program

COST

	Resident Tuition and Fees ($)	Non Resident Tuition and Fees ($)
Undergraduate	22,737	22,737
Medical school	23,675	23,675

COLLEGE
Florida Atlantic University

MEDICAL SCHOOL
Charles E. Schmidt College of Medicine

ADDRESS
Harriet L. Wilkes Honors College
Florida Atlantic University
Office of Admissions
5353 Parkside Drive
Jupiter, Florida 33458-2906
561-799-8646
www.fau.edu/divdept/honcol/admissions_med.htm
hcadmissions@fau.edu

NAME OF PROGRAM
Wilkes Medical Scholars Program

LENGTH OF PROGRAM
7 or 8 years

APPLICATION DEADLINE
February 1

INFORMATION ABOUT THE PROGRAM
Three applications are required for this program. Students must apply to the university, the Honors College, and the College of Medicine, the application for which includes two short essays. Students must be accepted into the honors program to be considered for the medical program. Students may major in many different areas within the liberal arts and sciences. Students may, with permission of the program, take four years for the undergraduate portion of the program to broaden their educational experiences.

Part of the curriculum includes medical electives and experiential programs during the year to prepare for medical school. Students are expected to participate in patient care experiences each summer of their undergraduate years. Students are also expected to keep a daily activity log of their enrichment and patient care experiences during their undergraduate years. Students who apply to other medical schools will lose their guaranteed spot at the medical school but may apply as regular applicants.

The program recommends that applicants have experience with patient interaction.

TRANSFER STUDENTS CONSIDERED
No

CITIZENSHIP REQUIREMENTS
U.S. citizen or permanent resident visa.

MINIMUM REQUIRED FACTORS IN SELECTION

CLASSES
Four years of English and math and one year each of biology and chemistry at a high school in the U.S.

GPA
4.3 weighted

SAT
1,400 critical reading and math; one or more SAT subject exams recommended but not required in one or more of math (level 2), biology, chemistry, and literature

ACT
32

ACCEPTANCES
No information provided

FACTORS REQUIRED TO CONTINUE IN PROGRAM
3.5 GPA each semester; science GPA after three years must be at least 3.5.

MCAT REQUIRED
Yes, minimum score above the 80th percentile

FINANCIAL AID
No special financial aid for students in the program

COST

	Resident Tuition and Fees ($)	Non Resident Tuition and Fees ($)
Undergraduate	6,039	21,595
Medical school	31,740	67,882

COLLEGE

University of Miami

MEDICAL SCHOOL

University of Miami Miller School of Medicine

ADDRESS

Office of Admissions
University of Miami
PO Box 248025
Coral Gables, Florida 33124-8025
305-284-4323
www.miami.edu/admission/index.php/undergraduate_admission
/academics/dual_degree_honors/honors_program_in_medicine/

NAME OF PROGRAM

Dual Degree Program in Medicine

LENGTH OF PROGRAM

7 or 8 years

APPLICATION DEADLINE

November 1 for both the undergraduate and supplemental
application

INFORMATION ABOUT THE PROGRAM

Personal factors—the student's maturity, common sense, empathy, interpersonal skills, freedom from parental influence, and compassion for others—are as important as academic factors in the admissions process. It is of critical importance to the admissions process that the student have self-initiated patient contact experiences. The supplemental application and all materials, including three recommendations, must be mailed together in one envelope by the November 1 deadline.

All students in the program are required to participate in a professionalism experience each semester they are enrolled in the undergraduate program. These experiences might include volunteering at health-related facilities, biomedical research, participation in area service organizations, or study abroad.

In 2015, Miami introduced a new short video application for selected students who were invited to the second step in the application process.

TRANSFER STUDENTS CONSIDERED

No

CITIZENSHIP REQUIREMENTS

U.S. citizen or permanent resident visa

MINIMUM REQUIRED FACTORS IN SELECTION

CLASSES

Four years of English and math, one year of biology, and one year of chemistry

GPA

Unweighted GPA of at least 3.75

SAT

1,400 on critical reading and math; SAT subject exams in math and one science, with minimum score of 600 on each test

ACT

32

ACCEPTANCES

About 15 to 20 students have typically been admitted to this program in recent years from over 200 applications. There is a slight preference for Florida residents.

FACTORS REQUIRED TO CONTINUE IN PROGRAM

Overall and science GPA of 3.7

MCAT REQUIRED

Yes, minimum score 30

FINANCIAL AID

No special financial aid for students in the program

COST

	Resident Tuition and Fees ($)	Non Resident Tuition and Fees ($)
Undergraduate	45,724	45,724
Medical school	37,163	42,626

COLLEGE

Augusta University

MEDICAL SCHOOL

Medical College of Georgia

ADDRESS

Augusta University
1120 15th Street
Augusta, Georgia 30912
404-809-8186
www.gru.edu/colleges/scimath/biology/bs-md-dmd.php
scholars@gru.edu

NAME OF PROGRAM

Medical Scholars Program

LENGTH OF PROGRAM

7 years

APPLICATION DEADLINE

November 15

INFORMATION ABOUT THE PROGRAM

Students in the program major in Cell and Molecular Biology in the College of Science and Mathematics. Students will complete their BS degree after their first year at the Medical College of Georgia.

There are two applications required, including application to the college and application to the program. A supplemental essay, letters of recommendation, and résumé are also required as part of the application.

TRANSFER STUDENTS CONSIDERED

No

CITIZENSHIP REQUIREMENTS

U.S. citizen or permanent resident visa. Preference is given to Georgia residents.

MINIMUM REQUIRED FACTORS IN SELECTION

CLASSES

No requirement specified

GPA

Unweighted GPA of at least 3.7

SAT

1,400 on critical reading and math

ACT

32

ACCEPTANCES

No information provided

FACTORS REQUIRED TO CONTINUE IN PROGRAM

Minimum cumulative and science GPA of 3.5 the first year, 3.6 the second year, and 3.7 the third year

MCAT REQUIRED

Yes, a minimum score no less than the prior year's national mean

FINANCIAL AID

No special financial aid given, although students are encouraged to apply for institutional scholarships.

COST

	Resident Tuition and Fees ($)	Non Resident Tuition and Fees ($)
Undergraduate	8,478	27,144
Medical school	34,896	56,716

COLLEGE
Mercer University

MEDICAL SCHOOL
Mercer University School of Medicine

ADDRESS
Mercer University
1501 Mercer University Drive
Macon, Georgia 31207
800-637-2378
https://medicine.mercer.edu/admissions/md
/enhancement-programs/guaranteed/

NAME OF PROGRAM
Guaranteed Admission Program

LENGTH OF PROGRAM
8 years

APPLICATION DEADLINE
December 1

INFORMATION ABOUT THE PROGRAM
There is a three-part application process. Hard copies of the pdf application much be mailed to the Mercer undergraduate college, and an email copy of the application must be sent to the program director. A minimum of two letters of reference are required including at least one from a science or math teacher and at least one character reference letter.

TRANSFER STUDENTS CONSIDERED
No

CITIZENSHIP REQUIREMENTS
U.S. citizen or permanent resident visa. Must be Georgia resident since January 1, 2013.

MINIMUM REQUIRED FACTORS IN SELECTION

CLASSES
No requirement specified

GPA
Unweighted GPA of at least 3.7

SAT
1,300, critical reading and math

ACT
29

ACCEPTANCES
Up to 10 students are admitted into the program each year.

FACTORS REQUIRED TO CONTINUE IN PROGRAM
Minimum cumulative and science GPA of 3.0 the end of first year, 3.25 the end of second year, and 3.5 the end of third year

MCAT REQUIRED
Yes, a minimum overall percentile rank of 67 and minimum percentile rank of 50 on the biological section of the new MCAT

FINANCIAL AID
No special financial aid given

COST

	Resident Tuition and Fees ($)	Non Resident Tuition and Fees ($)
Undergraduate	34,150	34,150
Medical school	41,457	41,457

COLLEGE

University of Hawaiʻi at Manoa

MEDICAL SCHOOL

John A. Burns School of Medicine

ADDRESS

University of Hawaiʻi at Manoa
Office of Admissions
2600 Campus Road, Room 001
Honolulu, Hawaiʻi 96822-2385
808-692-0892
www.manoa.hawaii.edu/admissions/undergrad/early_admissions/
uhmanoa.admissions@hawaii.edu

NAME OF PROGRAM

Doctor of Medicine Early Acceptance Program

LENGTH OF PROGRAM

8 years

APPLICATION DEADLINE

December 1

INFORMATION ABOUT THE PROGRAM

Students in the program will be part of the honors program at the college and will participate in summer clinical, research, and service internships. Volunteering and physician shadowing are part of the program requirements, as well as conducting research and completing a senior honors project.

Students will also have early interaction with faculty from the medical school. There are several study abroad programs available for students in the program, and fourth year medical students will have the opportunity for medical study abroad.

Students who demonstrate a commitment to serve in Hawaiʻi upon completion of the program are especially desirable candidates.

There are two applications required, including application to the college and application to the program. A supplemental essay, letters of recommendation, and résumé are also required as part of the application.

TRANSFER STUDENTS CONSIDERED

No

CITIZENSHIP REQUIREMENTS

U.S. citizen or permanent resident visa. Must also be a resident of Hawaiʻi.

MINIMUM REQUIRED FACTORS IN SELECTION

CLASSES

Pre-calculus, biology, chemistry, and physics must be completed or in progress. Students are expected to have AP credits.

GPA

Unweighted GPA of at least 3.8

SAT

1,800

ACT

27; writing section is required

ACCEPTANCES

A maximum of 10 new students are accepted each year.

FACTORS REQUIRED TO CONTINUE IN PROGRAM

3.5 cumulative GPA and 3.4 science GPA; maintain full-time status in the honors program

MCAT REQUIRED

Yes, minimum score of 509 on the new MCAT with no lower than 126 in any section or a 510 with no section lower than 125

FINANCIAL AID

Undergraduate tuition covers all four years of undergraduate education for students in the program.

COST

	Resident Tuition and Fees ($)	Non Resident Tuition and Fees ($)
Undergraduate	0	not applicable
Medical school	34,896	not applicable

Northwestern University
Northwestern University Feinberg School of Medicine
Associate Dean for Medical Education
Office of Admission and Financial Aid Northwestern University
1801 Hinman Avenue
Evanston, Illinois 60204-3060
312-503-8915
www.feinberg.northwestern.edu/education/degree-programs/hpme/
hpme@northwestern.edu
Honors Program in Medical Education (HPME)
7 or 8 years
December 1 for request for HPME application; January 1 for submission of application
Although often listed as a seven-year program, HPME encourages its students to consider spending eight years in the program. The goal of the program is to train the best students for a career in medicine while reducing the stress often associated with medical school applications. Students are encouraged to challenge themselves during their undergraduate years in an effort to develop personally and professionally.

As undergraduates, students may attend the Weinberg College of Arts, the School of Communication, or the McCormick School of Engineering at Northwestern. The courses they take depend on which undergraduate school they attend.

Students are provided with regular counseling to discuss the various options to them as undergraduates. There is a strong mentoring program available as part of the HPME program. There are also programs available where students can earn a PhD or a master's in public health (MPH). A summer research program is available to interested students after the first year of medical school.

This is a non-binding program and students are allowed to apply to other medical schools.
No

CITIZENSHIP REQUIREMENTS

International students accepted

MINIMUM REQUIRED FACTORS IN SELECTION

CLASSES

Four years of math (one year of calculus including differential and integral calculus are required before beginning HPME; if this is not offered at your high school, you must take the course before entering Northwestern); one year of chemistry (AP chemistry is highly recommended, and students will take a placement test the summer before starting the program if they haven't taken AP chemistry); one year of physics; one year of biology; four years of English; two years of foreign language (three to four years of the same language preferred)

GPA

No minimum but students are typically in top five percent of high school class

SAT

No minimum, but averages for accepted students are critical reading, 760; math, 785; writing, 772; subject tests in chemistry and math level 2 are required; no minimum, but averages for accepted students are chemistry, 770; and math level 2, 794

ACT

No minimum, but average is 35; average writing is 10

ACCEPTANCES

No information provided

FACTORS REQUIRED TO CONTINUE IN PROGRAM

Students are required to have a minimum 3.2 GPA in sciences courses and a minimum 3.4 GPA in overall academic courses.

MCAT REQUIRED

No

FINANCIAL AID

Northwestern meets one hundred percent of the demonstrated need for a student's undergraduate education. Northwestern also has financial aid available for medical school students.

COST

	Resident Tuition and Fees ($)	Non Resident Tuition and Fees ($)
Undergraduate	49,082	49,082
Medical school	53,947	53,947

COLLEGE

University of Illinois at Chicago

MEDICAL SCHOOL

University of Illinois at Chicago College of Medicine

ADDRESS

Assistant Director Academic Affairs/
Special Scholarship Programs
University of Illinois at Chicago
2506 University Hall, M/C 115
601 S. Morgan Street
Chicago, Illinois 60607-7100
312-355-2477
http://gppa.uic.edu/
gppauic@uic.edu

NAME OF PROGRAM

Guaranteed Professional Programs Admissions (GPPA)

LENGTH OF PROGRAM

8 years

APPLICATION DEADLINE

December 1

INFORMATION ABOUT THE PROGRAM

Students in this program are also required to apply to and participate in the Honors College of the university. This provides some
advantages in the way of services and facilities. An honors college interview is required. Students are encouraged to explore a
wide variety of majors and interests as well-rounded and cultured
students. While in the program, students must complete an independent study project, which includes a presentation. There are
several professionalism courses offered by the college of medicine
that students are required to attend.

The program places special emphasis on professionalism, integrity, and compassion for the human spirit.

Placement in medical school will be done at random in one
of four locations: Chicago, Peoria, Rockford, and Urbana–Cham-
paign. Location assignments will be made known at time of admission. Students may apply to medical schools outside the program.

TRANSFER STUDENTS CONSIDERED

No

CITIZENSHIP REQUIREMENTS

U.S. citizen or permanent resident visa; must also be Illinois resident

MINIMUM REQUIRED FACTORS IN SELECTION

CLASSES

No specific requirement

GPA

Average admitted student was in the top two percent of high school class.

SAT

1,240 critical reading and math

ACT

28; average admitted score was between 33 and 34.

ACCEPTANCES

Approximately 10 percent of applicants are admitted; an average of 50 students enter the program each year.

FACTORS REQUIRED TO CONTINUE IN PROGRAM

3.5 GPA, maintaining status in the Honors College, completion of required courses related to the medical profession, and completion of an independent study seminar project and presentation

MCAT REQUIRED

Yes; must earn score of at least the average of the matriculating students into the College of Medicine in the year prior to expected entry; it may be retaken up to three times.

FINANCIAL AID

In addition to regular financial aid, students admitted to the program are also considered for the Chancellor's GPPA Excellence Award of tuition and a portion of fees, renewable for the four years of undergraduate college.

COST

	Resident Tuition and Fees ($)	Non Resident Tuition and Fees ($)
Undergraduate	9,526	not applicable
Medical school	35,442	not applicable

COLLEGE
Indiana State University

MEDICAL SCHOOL
Indiana University School of Medicine–Terre Haute

ADDRESS
Stalker Hall 205
Indiana State University
200 North Seventh Street
Terre Haute, Indiana 47809-9989
812-237-8633
www.indstate.edu/cas/pre-professional-programs
/bmd-rural-health-program/overview
preprof@indstate.edu

NAME OF PROGRAM
B/MD Rural Health Program

LENGTH OF PROGRAM
8 years

APPLICATION DEADLINE
December 15

INFORMATION ABOUT THE PROGRAM
This specialized program is only open to residents of rural Indiana. Students may major in any undergraduate degree and are a part of the university honors program. Students in the program have interaction with faculty of the school of medicine including the opportunity to participate in a mini-medical school. Students also have summer internship experiences with rural physicians and undergraduate research experience.

TRANSFER STUDENTS CONSIDERED
No

CITIZENSHIP REQUIREMENTS
U.S. citizen or permanent resident visa; must reside in rural Indiana

MINIMUM REQUIRED FACTORS IN SELECTION

CLASSES

No specific requirement

GPA

3.5 unweighted

SAT

1,200 critical reading and math

ACT

27

ACCEPTANCES

Approximately 10 new students matriculate each year.

FACTORS REQUIRED TO CONTINUE IN PROGRAM

Undergraduate minimum GPA of 3.5

MCAT REQUIRED

Yes; score must be at least equal to the mean score of the previous year's entering class.

FINANCIAL AID

Students in program receive full tuition waiver for undergraduate study.

COST

	Resident Tuition and Fees ($)	Non Resident Tuition and Fees ($)
Undergraduate	0	not applicable
Medical school	33,474	not applicable

COLLEGE
University of Evansville

MEDICAL SCHOOL
Indiana University School of Medicine–Evansville

ADDRESS
Koch Center for Engineering and Science
Room 326
University of Evansville
Evansville, Indiana 47722
812-488-1077
https://www.evansville.edu/majors/BtoMD/
km123@evansville.edu

NAME OF PROGRAM
Baccalaureate to Doctor of Medicine (B/MD) Program

LENGTH OF PROGRAM
8 years

APPLICATION DEADLINE
December 1 undergraduate; December 15 medical school

INFORMATION ABOUT THE PROGRAM
This program is intended to increase the number of physicians in southern and southwestern Indiana. Four letters of recommendation are required from a teacher, guidance counselor, school principal, and an additional unrelated individual. Students may major in any undergraduate degree.

Students also have access to enrichment experiences including early clinical opportunities, community service, and undergraduate research.

TRANSFER STUDENTS CONSIDERED
No

CITIZENSHIP REQUIREMENTS
U.S. citizen or permanent resident visa; Indiana residents only

MINIMUM REQUIRED FACTORS IN SELECTION

CLASSES
No specific requirement

GPA
Approximate average of 4.0

SAT
1,920 critical reading and math and writing

ACT
29

ACCEPTANCES
Approximately 8 new students are accepted each year.

FACTORS REQUIRED TO CONTINUE IN PROGRAM
GPA of 3.0 for the first 31 undergraduate hours and a cumulative of 3.5 from there on

MCAT REQUIRED
Yes; score must be at least equal to the average of the previous year's entering class.

FINANCIAL AID
Students in program receive strong consideration for merit scholarships for the undergraduate years.

COST

	Resident Tuition and Fees ($)	Non Resident Tuition and Fees ($)
Undergraduate	32,946	not applicable
Medical school	33,474	not applicable

COLLEGE
University of Louisville

MEDICAL SCHOOL
University of Louisville School of Medicine

ADDRESS
Office of Admissions
University of Louisville
Houchens Building, Room 150
2211 S. Brook Street
Louisville, Kentucky 40208-1874
502-852-6531
https://louisville.edu/admissions/aid/gep/gems
admitme@louisville.edu

NAME OF PROGRAM
Guaranteed Entrance to Medical School (GEMS)

LENGTH OF PROGRAM
8 years

APPLICATION DEADLINE
December 15

INFORMATION ABOUT THE PROGRAM
Students in the program will have hands-on experience with the medical school, including physician shadowing and enhanced opportunities for research and professional meetings. Applicants to the program need to provide an essay discussing their plans and goals for the future; two recommendation letters, including one from a principal or counselor, and one from a science teacher or math teacher.

TRANSFER STUDENTS CONSIDERED
No

CITIZENSHIP REQUIREMENTS
U.S. citizen or permanent resident visa; must also be a resident of Kentucky and attend high school in Kentucky

MINIMUM REQUIRED FACTORS IN SELECTION

CLASSES

No specific requirement

GPA

Unweighted GPA of at least 3.75; top five percent of high school class

SAT

1,360 critical reading and math

ACT

31

ACCEPTANCES

No information provided

FACTORS REQUIRED TO CONTINUE IN PROGRAM

3.4 cumulative GPA

MCAT REQUIRED

Yes; score at or above the national mean on each section of the test

FINANCIAL AID

No special financial aid for students in the program

COST

	Resident Tuition and Fees ($)	Non Resident Tuition and Fees ($)
Undergraduate	10,542	not applicable
Medical school	36,464	not applicable

COLLEGE
Boston University

MEDICAL SCHOOL
Boston University School of Medicine

ADDRESS
Boston University
Office of Undergraduate Admissions
121 Bay State Road
Boston, Massachusetts 02215-1714
617-353-2300
www.bu.edu/academics/cas/programs
/seven-year-liberal-arts-medical-education-program/
admissions@bu.edu

NAME OF PROGRAM
Seven-Year Liberal Arts/Medical Education Program

LENGTH OF PROGRAM
7 years

APPLICATION DEADLINE
November 15

INFORMATION ABOUT THE PROGRAM
Students spend the first three years of the program studying at the College of Arts & Sciences. During this time they take pre-medical science courses as well as elective course in the humanities and social sciences. Students are also required to take a biology course and other elective courses during the second summer in the program. After completing the required undergraduate science courses in the first two years of the program, students may take modular medical courses in the third year of the program. Many of these modular courses are equivalent to first year medical school courses.

All students are also required to complete a minor in a discipline approved by the College of Arts & Sciences. Students are not allowed to apply to other medical schools and remain in the program.

TRANSFER STUDENTS CONSIDERED
No

CITIZENSHIP REQUIREMENTS
International students considered

MINIMUM REQUIRED FACTORS IN SELECTION

CLASSES

Four years English and math including one year of calculus, three years social sciences, three years foreign languages, one year biology, one year physics, one year of chemistry (AP chemistry recommended)

GPA

No specific GPA; typical successful applicants had a 3.9 GPA unweighted and were in the top one percent of their high school class.

SAT

No specific SAT; average SAT score of successful candidates was 2,274; subject tests are required in math level 2 and chemistry; subject test in a foreign language is recommended; average chemistry subject test score, 759; average math level 2 score, 778.

ACT

No specific requirement

ACCEPTANCES

Recently, approximately 25 new students have been admitted from an applicant pool of over 700.

FACTORS REQUIRED TO CONTINUE IN PROGRAM

3.2 GPA cumulative and in the sciences

MCAT REQUIRED

Yes; a minimum combined score at or above the 80th percentile is required

FINANCIAL AID

Need-based aid available for undergraduates; loans available for medical school students

COST

	Resident Tuition and Fees ($)	Non Resident Tuition and Fees ($)
Undergraduate	47,422	47,422
Medical school	53,894	53,894

COLLEGE
Northern Michigan University

MEDICAL SCHOOL
Wayne State University School of Medicine

ADDRESS
Director of Admissions
Northern Michigan University
1401 Presque Isle Avenue
Marquette, Michigan 49855-5305
906-227-2650
www.nmu.edu/preprofessional/node/24
admiss@nmu.edu

NAME OF PROGRAM
MedStart

LENGTH OF PROGRAM
8 years

APPLICATION DEADLINE
February 1. It is recommended that the undergraduate application be completed by mid-January.

INFORMATION ABOUT THE PROGRAM
Students must complete two applications, an application to the undergraduate college and an application to the program. Both applications must be completed by the deadline date.

The program emphasizes mentoring and research activities and includes early contact with faculty and students of the medical school. A number of activities are available for students in the pre-medical program at Northern Michigan University; students are expected to take advantage of the opportunities, including pre-professional clubs and hospital seminars. Freshmen are assigned a local physician to shadow, and they attend physician seminars.

Preference in admissions is given to students from medically underserved areas who have an interest in working as a primary care physician in such areas. Students are allowed to apply to other medical schools.

TRANSFER STUDENTS CONSIDERED
No

CITIZENSHIP REQUIREMENTS

U.S. citizen or permanent resident visa

MINIMUM REQUIRED FACTORS IN SELECTION

CLASSES

No specific requirement

GPA

3.5 in academic core courses; classes are weighted for AP/IB/honors courses

SAT

1,240 on critical reading and math

ACT

28

ACCEPTANCES

No information provided

FACTORS REQUIRED TO CONTINUE IN PROGRAM

GPA of 3.5 cumulative and in science courses, including grades of B or higher on all courses required by school of medicine; active participation in the college's premedical activities; ongoing involvement with health-related volunteer work

MCAT REQUIRED

Yes; minimum score 24 with at least an 8 in biological sciences

FINANCIAL AID

Students in the program are guaranteed scholarship support at the college.

COST

	Resident Tuition and Fees ($)	Non Resident Tuition and Fees ($)
Undergraduate	9,556	14,956
Medical school	33,057	65,346

COLLEGE

Wayne State University

MEDICAL SCHOOL

Wayne State University School of Medicine

ADDRESS

Program Coordinator
Irvin D. Reid Honors College
Wayne State University
2100 Undergraduate Library
Detroit, Michigan 48202-3900
313-577-3030
http://honors.wayne.edu/future/waynemeddirect.php
honors@wayne.edu

NAME OF PROGRAM

Wayne Med-Direct

LENGTH OF PROGRAM

8 years

APPLICATION DEADLINE

January 15

INFORMATION ABOUT THE PROGRAM

The program emphasizes mentoring and research activities and
includes early contact with faculty and students of the medical
school. A number of activities are available for students in the
program, and students are expected to take advantage of the
opportunities.

Preference is given to students from disadvantaged socio-
economic backgrounds who are interested in studying health
disparities.

TRANSFER STUDENTS CONSIDERED

No

CITIZENSHIP REQUIREMENTS

U.S. citizen or permanent resident visa

MINIMUM REQUIRED FACTORS IN SELECTION

CLASSES

No specific requirement

GPA

3.5

SAT

1,340 on critical reading and math

ACT

30

ACCEPTANCES

Up to 10 students per year are admitted to the program.

FACTORS REQUIRED TO CONTINUE IN PROGRAM

Good standing in the honors college with a 3.3 GPA for the first year and a 3.5 GPA thereafter; 3.5 GPA in biology, chemistry, physics, and math, with no grade less than a B; participation in Med Direct seminars, physician shadowing experiences, volunteer work in a health care field, and various aspects of the Med Direct program. Students must graduate with university honors, including a senior thesis and senior seminar.

MCAT REQUIRED

Yes. Current numbers are being determined, but in the past students were required to score 10 on each section and minimum total of 30.

FINANCIAL AID

Students admitted to Med Direct are provided paid undergraduate tuition, room, and board, as well as medical school tuition.

COST

	Resident Tuition and Fees ($)	Non Resident Tuition and Fees ($)
Undergraduate	0	0
Medical school	0	0

COLLEGE

University of Missouri Kansas City

MEDICAL SCHOOL

University of Missouri Kansas City School of Medicine

ADDRESS

UMKC School of Medicine
Council on Selection
2411 Holmes
Kansas City, Missouri 64108-2792
816-235-1870
www.med.umkc.edu/bamd/
medicine@umkc.edu

NAME OF PROGRAM

Six Year B.A./M.D. Program

LENGTH OF PROGRAM

6 years

APPLICATION DEADLINE

November 1

INFORMATION ABOUT THE PROGRAM

This program is one of the largest in the country. The majority of students in the medical school come through the BA/MD program. This is a year-round program, and the medical school classes and undergraduate classes are combined during all six years.

During the first two years of the program, three quarters of the student's time is spent on the arts and science education required to fulfill the BA degree requirements; one quarter of the time is spent on medical school courses. During this time students are assigned primary care physicians to mentor the students in the fundamentals of medicine. During the last four years of the program this ratio is reversed, with three quarters of the time spent on medical school courses and one quarter of the time on courses to fulfill the BA degree requirements.

There is an emphasis on medical humanities at the school of medicine; during year five or six the student spends a month gaining a broader appreciation of art, literature, and philosophy, while cultivating compassion and empathy.

During years three to six, the student is assigned to a docent unit, made up of a senior student, a clinical pharmacologist, and other health care professionals. These units provide a small group learning environment, and each unit spends a half day per week providing outpatient care in local clinics.

Fifth year students spend one month in a rural Missouri preceptorship to provide experience in addressing health care concerns in a non-urban primary care clinic as well as experience with the business operation of a small town physician.

TRANSFER STUDENTS CONSIDERED

Yes, for students with fewer than twenty-four hours of post–high school college credit

CITIZENSHIP REQUIREMENTS

U.S. citizen or permanent resident visa; students must also have graduated from a U.S. accredited high school

MINIMUM REQUIRED FACTORS IN SELECTION

CLASSES

Four years of English and math, three years of science (including one year of biology and one year of chemistry), three years of social studies, two years of a single foreign language, and one year of fine arts

GPA

3.0; average GPA of accepted Missouri residents is 3.80 and of out-of-state residents is 3.85

SAT

1,090 math and critical reading. Writing section is not considered. Accepted for out-of-state residents but ACT preferred; average for out-of-state residents is 1,380.

ACT

24. Writing section is not considered. ACT required for Missouri residents; average ACT for accepted in-state residents is 30; average for out-of-state residents is 31

ACCEPTANCES

This is one of the largest programs in the country taking 100–115 new students per year. Over half (60–65) of the admitted students are Missouri residents; 30–35 students are typically admitted from regional states (Arkansas, Kansas, Illinois, Nebraska, and Oklahoma); and 10–15 students are from elsewhere.

FACTORS REQUIRED TO CONTINUE IN PROGRAM

Minimum cumulative 2.7 GPA

MCAT REQUIRED

No

FINANCIAL AID

No special financial aid for students in the program

COST

	Resident Tuition and Fees ($)	Non Resident Tuition and Fees ($)
Undergraduate	9,553	22,714
Medical school	30,514	59,232

COLLEGE

Washington University in St. Louis

MEDICAL SCHOOL

Washington University in St. Louis School of Medicine

ADDRESS

Undergraduate Admissions
Washington University in St. Louis
One Brookings Drive
St. Louis, Missouri 63130-4862
800-638-0700; 314-935-6000
http://uscholars.wustl.edu
uscholars@wustl.edu

NAME OF PROGRAM

University Scholars Program in Medicine

LENGTH OF PROGRAM

8 years

APPLICATION DEADLINE

January 15 for undergraduate and supplement application

INFORMATION ABOUT THE PROGRAM

Students may major in any subject and are welcome to engage in
study abroad programs. Students in the program often engage in
research if they desire, and this is often with faculty members of
the medical school. Program participants have the opportunity
for doctor shadowing and personalized pre-professional advising.
Students in the program are allowed to apply to other medical
schools.

Students considering this program should be aware of several
factors. The requirements for students to advance to the medical school are the most stringent of any BS/MD program. Participants are required to maintain a high GPA and have a very high
MCAT score. It is also our experience that for admittance to the
program, students should show particular interest in Washington
University, including visiting the campus if at all possible.

TRANSFER STUDENTS CONSIDERED

No

CITIZENSHIP REQUIREMENTS

International students considered

MINIMUM REQUIRED FACTORS IN SELECTION

None specified

ACCEPTANCES

In past years, approximately 10 new students have been admitted per year.

FACTORS REQUIRED TO CONTINUE IN PROGRAM

3.8 GPA overall

MCAT REQUIRED

Yes; minimum score of 516 required

FINANCIAL AID

There are no scholarships specified for students in the program. Washington University does meet one hundred percent of the need of admitted students for undergraduate study. The medical school does have need-based scholarships and loans. There are also merit-based scholarships available for the medical school.

COST

	Resident Tuition and Fees ($)	Non Resident Tuition and Fees ($)
Undergraduate	48,093	48,093
Medical school	54,050	54,050

COLLEGE

Chadron State College; Wayne State College

MEDICAL SCHOOL

University of Nebraska Medical Center

ADDRESS

Health Professions Office
Chadron State College
1000 Main Street
Chadron, Nebraska 69337
308-432-6278
www.csc.edu/sci/rhop/
hpoffice@csc.edu

Health Professions Office
Wayne State College
1111 Main Street
Wayne, Nebraska 68787
402-375-7329
www.wsc.edu/rhop/
preprof@wsc.edu

www.unmc.edu/studentservices/rse/enrichment
/rural-health-enrichment-programs/rhop/index.html

NAME OF PROGRAM

Rural Health Opportunities Program

LENGTH OF PROGRAM

8 years

APPLICATION DEADLINE

November 15

INFORMATION ABOUT THE PROGRAM

The purpose of this program is to educate students from rural Nebraska who wish to return to practice medicine in rural areas of the state. Non-traditional students are encouraged to apply. Students may apply to only one of the programs.

TRANSFER STUDENTS CONSIDERED

No

CITIZENSHIP REQUIREMENTS

U.S. citizen or permanent resident visa; must be a resident of rural Nebraska and a graduate of a Nebraska high school

MINIMUM REQUIRED FACTORS IN SELECTION

CLASSES

Strongly recommend four years of English, three years of math, and one year each of biology, chemistry, and physics

GPA

No specific requirement

SAT

No specific requirement

ACT

24

ACCEPTANCES

There are position openings for 4 students at Chadron and 5 students at Wayne.

FACTORS REQUIRED TO CONTINUE IN PROGRAM

3.5 overall and a C or better in every class

MCAT REQUIRED

Yes; minimum score 24

FINANCIAL AID

Students in the program will receive tuition waiver for up to sixteen credits per term during their undergraduate years.

COST

	Resident Tuition and Fees ($)	Non Resident Tuition and Fees ($)
Undergraduate	0	not applicable
Medical school	29,194	not applicable

COLLEGE
University of Nevada, Las Vegas; University of Nevada, Reno

MEDICAL SCHOOL
University of Nevada School of Medicine

ADDRESS
University of Nevada School of Medicine Las Vegas
Admin Building, Suite 504
2040 West Charleston Boulevard
Las Vegas, Nevada 89102

Pennington Medical Education Building
1664 N. Virginia Street
Reno, Nevada 89557-0357
775-784-6063

http://medicine.nevada.edu/admissions/admissions
/special-programs/bs-md
bsmd@medicine.nevada.edu

NAME OF PROGRAM
BS-MD Accelerated Program

LENGTH OF PROGRAM
7 years

APPLICATION DEADLINE
January 22

INFORMATION ABOUT THE PROGRAM
Both of the undergraduate colleges associated with this program
may have up to six students admitted into the program. Students
must select which college they wish to apply to before applying to
the program. Research and clinical experience is expected of all
students in the program during their undergraduate years. Students must select from a limited number of science majors. At the
start of the program, students are paired with a medical student
mentor.

TRANSFER STUDENTS CONSIDERED
No

CITIZENSHIP REQUIREMENTS
U.S. citizen or permanent resident visa; Nevada residency; must
also attend a Nevada high school for a minimum of two years and
graduate from a Nevada high school

MINIMUM REQUIRED FACTORS IN SELECTION

CLASSES

No specific requirement

GPA

3.7 unweighted or top ten percent of high school class

SAT

1,270 on critical reading and math

ACT

29

ACCEPTANCES

Space for 12 new students each year

FACTORS REQUIRED TO CONTINUE IN PROGRAM

3.5 overall and science GPA

MCAT REQUIRED

Yes; minimum score 28 with no sub-score below 7

FINANCIAL AID

No special financial aid for students in the program

COST

	Resident Tuition and Fees ($)	Non Resident Tuition and Fees ($)
Undergraduate	7,012	not applicable
Medical school	25,110	not applicable

COLLEGE

Caldwell College

MEDICAL SCHOOL

Rutgers Biomedical and Health Sciences

ADDRESS

Caldwell College
120 Bloomfield Avenue
Caldwell, New Jersey 07006-5310
973-618-3000
www.caldwell.edu/academics/health-professions
/affiliation-programs
admissions@caldwell.edu

NAME OF PROGRAM

Health Professions Affiliation Program Medicine

LENGTH OF PROGRAM

7 or 8 years

APPLICATION DEADLINE

January 15

INFORMATION ABOUT THE PROGRAM

This is one of eight programs associated with the Rutgers Biomedical and Health Sciences. The medical school was formerly known as New Jersey Medical School. Students can major in any topic.

TRANSFER STUDENTS CONSIDERED

No

CITIZENSHIP REQUIREMENTS

U.S. citizen or permanent resident visa

MINIMUM REQUIRED FACTORS IN SELECTION

CLASSES

No specific requirements

GPA

3.50 unweighted; top 10 percent of high school class

SAT

1,400 critical reading and math

ACT

32

FACTORS REQUIRED TO CONTINUE IN PROGRAM

3.5 overall GPA each semester; grades of B or better in all premedical classes

MCAT REQUIRED

Yes, but it will not be used in determining matriculation to the medical school.

FINANCIAL AID

No special financial aid for students in the program

COST

	Resident Tuition and Fees ($)	Non Resident Tuition and Fees ($)
Undergraduate	31,400	31,400
Medical school	42,887	63,802

COLLEGE

The College of New Jersey

MEDICAL SCHOOL

Rutgers Biomedical and Health Sciences

ADDRESS

Chairman, Medical Careers Committee,
The College of New Jersey
PO Box 7718
Ewing, New Jersey 08628-0718
609-771-2021
http://biology.pages.tcnj.edu/biology-programs
/medical-careers/7-year-medical-program/
medcar@tcnj.edu

NAME OF PROGRAM

Combined BS/MD 7-Year Program

LENGTH OF PROGRAM

7 years

APPLICATION DEADLINE

December 1

INFORMATION ABOUT THE PROGRAM

This is one of eight programs associated with the Rutgers Biomedical and Health Sciences. Students in the program spend three years at the college and must major in an approved major—biology, chemistry, English, philosophy, biomedical engineering, math, economics, physics, or history. If students have earned college credit through AP courses or early college credit, they may also apply for mechanical or electrical engineering as a major. No additional time is required at the college other than a summer research project that must be completed before the first year of medical school.

Students with high academic achievement and a record of community service may be asked to interview with a medical career advisor at the college. Telephone interviews are allowed only for students living far from New Jersey. If that interview is favorable you will then be asked to interview with the medical school admissions office at the medical school. This interview must be in person. Typically, half or more of the students in the eight BS/MD programs associated with Rutgers Biomedical and Health Sciences come from The College of New Jersey. Students in the program are allowed to apply out to other medical schools during the fourth year of the program, but they will then lose their guaranteed acceptance to the medical school.

TRANSFER STUDENTS CONSIDERED

No

CITIZENSHIP REQUIREMENTS

U.S. citizen or permanent resident visa. Students who do not have U.S. citizenship or permanent resident status may apply as long as they qualify for citizenship or permanent resident status before starting at the medical school.

MINIMUM REQUIRED FACTORS IN SELECTION

CLASSES

No specific requirement

GPA

Top five percent or have a GPA of 4.5 or 95 percent, depending on the school. If high school does not rank, the admissions office will call the head guidance counselor of your school to evaluate your ranking and transcript. Average GPA of accepted students is 4.72.

SAT

1,500 critical reading and math. Average score of accepted students is 1,534. SAT subject tests are optional, but of those submitted, the average score was 730.

ACT

Now accepted; must be 35

ACCEPTANCES

Approximately 400 students apply each year; 80 are interviewed by the medical school for 20 spots.

FACTORS REQUIRED TO CONTINUE IN PROGRAM

3.5 cumulative and science GPA in approved major each semester; grade of B or better in each of the basic science courses required by the medical school; no grade below a C in any course. Students must engage in a research experience before beginning the medical school.

MCAT REQUIRED

Yes; no minimum score required, but students are encouraged to achieve at least the national mean, which in the past was a 31.

FINANCIAL AID

No special financial aid for students in the program

COST

	Resident Tuition and Fees ($)	Non Resident Tuition and Fees ($)
Undergraduate	15,446	26,378
Medical school	42,887	63,802

COLLEGE
Drew University

MEDICAL SCHOOL
Rutgers Biomedical and Health Sciences

ADDRESS
College Admissions
Drew University
36 Madison Avenue
Madison, New Jersey 07940-1434
973-408-3739
www.drew.edu/undergraduate/what-you-learn/pre-med
/dual-degree
cadm@drew.edu

NAME OF PROGRAM
Dual-Degree Program (B.A./M.D.) in Medicine

LENGTH OF PROGRAM
7 years

APPLICATION DEADLINE
November 1

INFORMATION ABOUT THE PROGRAM
This is one of eight programs associated with the Rutgers Biomedical and Health Sciences. Students in the program may major
in any subject while at Drew. In addition to major requirements, a
student must meet general education requirements and take basic
pre-medical courses.

An in-person interview with Drew University is required and
should be held by December 1. The applications of qualified candidates will then be sent to the medical school, where students will
be selected for in-person interviews at the medical school. A student may apply to other medical schools but will lose their guaranteed spot if they do so.

TRANSFER STUDENTS CONSIDERED
No

CITIZENSHIP REQUIREMENTS
U.S. citizen or permanent resident visa

MINIMUM REQUIRED FACTORS IN SELECTION

CLASSES
No specific requirement

GPA
3.8 unweighted GPA

SAT
1,400 critical reading and math. SAT subject tests in math and science are optional but recommended.

ACT
32

ACCEPTANCES
Typically receive 60–100 applications for 5–10 spots

FACTORS REQUIRED TO CONTINUE IN PROGRAM
Students must carry at least fourteen credit hours per semester and maintain a 3.4 GPA overall and for science courses each semester. No grade lower than a B– is allowed in one of the required pre-medical courses.

MCAT REQUIRED
Yes; no minimum score required

FINANCIAL AID
No special financial aid for students in the program

COST

	Resident Tuition and Fees ($)	Non Resident Tuition and Fees ($)
Undergraduate	45,552	45,552
Medical school	42,887	63,802

COLLEGE
Montclair State University

MEDICAL SCHOOL
Rutgers Biomedical and Health Sciences

ADDRESS
Health Professions Committee
Department of Biology
Montclair State University
1 Normal Avenue
Montclair, New Jersey 07043-1699
973-655-4397
www.montclair.edu/csam/health-careers/combined-bs-md/
msuadm@mail.montclair.edu

NAME OF PROGRAM
Health Careers Program Combined BS/MD Program

LENGTH OF PROGRAM
8 years

APPLICATION DEADLINE
December 15

INFORMATION ABOUT THE PROGRAM
This is one of eight programs associated with the Rutgers Biomedical and Health Sciences. This program is for students from financially and educationally disadvantaged backgrounds. Students major in biology, chemistry, biochemistry or molecular biology. An in-person interview at the college is offered to selected students. A parent or guardian must accompany the student to the interview. The student must show motivation, maturity, and an understanding of the demands of the medical profession during the interview. All students must participate in the honors program. Letters of recommendation are required from a teacher of math, a teacher of science, and an English teacher. The program will accept a maximum of five letters of recommendation. After the first interview, selected students are invited to interview with the medical school.

Summer enrichment activities are required.

TRANSFER STUDENTS CONSIDERED
No

CITIZENSHIP REQUIREMENTS
U.S. citizen or permanent resident visa and New Jersey resident

MINIMUM REQUIRED FACTORS IN SELECTION

CLASSES

Four years English, two years of the same foreign language, two years social studies, three years math through at least geometry, one year of biology with lab, one year of chemistry with lab, and three years of electives.

GPA

Top ten percent high school class and B average or above GPA and at least a B average in math and science

SAT

1,100 with at least 550 on both critical reading and math on a single test

ACT

Not accepted

FACTORS REQUIRED TO CONTINUE IN PROGRAM

GPA of 3.2 or better, minimum grade of B in required pre-med science courses; fulfillment of requirements of the honors curriculum; and participation in summer study or independent research at Rutgers Biomedical and Health Sciences

MCAT REQUIRED

Yes; no minimum score required but should be competitive

FINANCIAL AID

No special financial aid program for students in the program

COST

	Resident Tuition and Fees ($)	Non Resident Tuition and Fees ($)
Undergraduate	11,772	not applicable
Medical school	42,887	not applicable

COLLEGE
New Jersey Institute of Technology

MEDICAL SCHOOL
Rutgers Biomedical and Health Sciences

ADDRESS
Honors College
New Jersey Institute of Technology
University Heights
Newark, New Jersey 07102-1982
973-642-7664
http://honors.njit.edu/admission/pre-health-law/health.php
http://honors.njit.edu/academics/acceleratedprograms
/PreHealthCareers.php
Darshan@njit.edu

NAME OF PROGRAM
Accelerated Medical Program

LENGTH OF PROGRAM
7 years

APPLICATION DEADLINE
November 15

INFORMATION ABOUT THE PROGRAM
This is one of eight programs associated with the Rutgers Biomedical and Health Sciences. Students applying to this program
are first required to interview and be accepted into the Honors
College. Those accepted into the Honors College then have their
application sent to the medical school for review. Applicants are
expected to show they have knowledge of the medical field through
research or volunteer activities. The curriculum at the Honors
College includes research and professional exploration. Students
may choose any major, but preferred majors are biology; biomedical engineering; biochemistry; biophysics; mathematics; or science, technology, and society (STS).

TRANSFER STUDENTS CONSIDERED
No

CITIZENSHIP REQUIREMENTS
U.S. citizen or permanent resident visa by start of professional
program

MINIMUM REQUIRED FACTORS IN SELECTION

CLASSES

No specific requirement

GPA

Top ten percent of high school class

SAT

1,450 critical reading and math in one sitting; typical score is 1,500

ACT

33

FACTORS REQUIRED TO CONTINUE IN PROGRAM

Students must maintain a 3.4 GPA each semester in the program; minimum B grade in all required science courses

MCAT REQUIRED

Yes; no minimum score required

FINANCIAL AID

Students admitted to program receive a scholarship that covers the full cost of attendance.

COST

	Resident Tuition and Fees ($)	Non Resident Tuition and Fees ($)
Undergraduate	0	0
Medical school	42,887	63,802

COLLEGE
The Richard Stockton College of New Jersey

MEDICAL SCHOOL
Rutgers Biomedical and Health Sciences

ADDRESS
The Richard Stockton College of New Jersey
Jimmie Leeds Road
Pomona, New Jersey 08240-0088
609-642-7664
http://intraweb.stockton.edu/eyos/admissions_home/content
/images/2011docs/dual%20degree%20health%20info.pdf

NAME OF PROGRAM
Dual Degree Health Professions Program

LENGTH OF PROGRAM
7 years

APPLICATION DEADLINE
December 15

INFORMATION ABOUT THE PROGRAM
This is one of eight programs associated with the Rutgers Biomedical and Health Sciences. There is a supplemental application
required for this program in addition to the regular application for
admission. Students major in biology.

TRANSFER STUDENTS CONSIDERED
No

CITIZENSHIP REQUIREMENTS
U.S. citizen or permanent resident visa

MINIMUM REQUIRED FACTORS IN SELECTION

CLASSES

Four years of English, three years of science, three years of math

GPA

Top ten percent of high school class

SAT

700 each in the critical reading and math sections from one test

ACT

Not accepted

FACTORS REQUIRED TO CONTINUE IN PROGRAM

Minimum 3.0 GPA while at Richard Stockton and a minimum grade of B in each course required for admission to the medical school; no grade below a B is accepted for required courses and classes cannot be repeated to earn a higher grade

MCAT REQUIRED

Yes, no minimum score

FINANCIAL AID

No special financial aid for students in the program

COST

	Resident Tuition and Fees ($)	Non Resident Tuition and Fees ($)
Undergraduate	12,820	19,472
Medical school	42,878	63,802

COLLEGE

Rutgers–Newark College of Arts and Sciences

MEDICAL SCHOOL

Rutgers Biomedical and Health Sciences

ADDRESS

Office of Admissions-BA/MD Program
Rutgers University
249 University Avenue, Room 100
Newark, New Jersey 07102-1808
973-353-5205
www.ncas.rutgers.edu/office-dean-student-affairs
/bamd-program-umdnj-nwk-applying

NAME OF PROGRAM

BA/MD Program

LENGTH OF PROGRAM

7 years

APPLICATION DEADLINE

November 1

INFORMATION ABOUT THE PROGRAM

This is one of eight programs associated with Rutgers Biomedical and Health Sciences. All documents must be sent from high school guidance office of student in one packet. In addition to the application to the college, students must also complete a Rutgers University Self Reported Academic Record and a BA/MD portfolio. Interviews are first conducted by Rutgers, and if the student is recommended to the medical school, then the medical school may also schedule an interview. Students in this program can choose from six majors: English, biology, chemistry, economics, psychology, and history.

TRANSFER STUDENTS CONSIDERED

No

CITIZENSHIP REQUIREMENTS

U.S. citizen or permanent resident visa

MINIMUM REQUIRED FACTORS IN SELECTION

CLASSES

No specific requirement

GPA

Top ten percent of high school class

SAT

1,400 critical reading and math

ACT

32; writing section required

FACTORS REQUIRED TO CONTINUE IN PROGRAM

None listed

MCAT REQUIRED

Yes; no minimum score required

FINANCIAL AID

No special financial aid for students in the program

COST

	Resident Tuition and Fees ($)	Non Resident Tuition and Fees ($)
Undergraduate	14,000	28,890
Medical school	42,887	63,802

COLLEGE
Stevens Institute of Technology

MEDICAL SCHOOL
Rutgers Biomedical and Health Sciences

ADDRESS
Director of Honors Admissions Programs
Stevens Institute of Technology
Castle Point on Hudson
Hoboken, New Jersey 07030-5991
201-216-5163
www.stevens.edu/sit/admissions/academics/preprofessional.cfm

NAME OF PROGRAM
Accelerated Combined Degree Programs

LENGTH OF PROGRAM
7 years

APPLICATION DEADLINE
November 15

INFORMATION ABOUT THE PROGRAM
This is one of eight programs associated with Rutgers Biomedical and Health Sciences. Students in the program take a specific program of courses at Stevens that includes course overloads. Students major in chemical biology. An interview at Stevens is required, and you may also be asked to interview with the medical school.

TRANSFER STUDENTS CONSIDERED
No

CITIZENSHIP REQUIREMENTS
U.S. citizen or permanent resident visa

MINIMUM REQUIRED FACTORS IN SELECTION

CLASSES

Four years of English; four years of math through at least pre-calculus; one year each of biology, chemistry, and physics; AP biology and AP chemistry are recommended if available

GPA

Top ten percent of high school class

SAT

1,400 critical reading and math in one sitting; subject test in math, level 1 or 2, and chemistry or biology also required

ACT

No specific requirement

FACTORS REQUIRED TO CONTINUE IN PROGRAM

None listed

MCAT REQUIRED

Yes; no minimum required

FINANCIAL AID

No special financial aid for students in the program

COST

	Resident Tuition and Fees ($)	Non Resident Tuition and Fees ($)
Undergraduate	45,540	45,540
Medical school	42,887	63,802

COLLEGE

University of New Mexico

MEDICAL SCHOOL

University of New Mexico School of Medicine

ADDRESS

SOM Director, Combined BA/MD Program
1 University of New Mexico, MSC 09 5065
Albuquerque, New Mexico 87131-0001
505-925-4500
http://som.unm.edu/education/bamd/index.html
bamdas@unm.edu
HSC-Combinedbamd@salud.unm.edu

NAME OF PROGRAM

Combined BA/MD Program

LENGTH OF PROGRAM

8 years

APPLICATION DEADLINE

Second Friday in November

INFORMATION ABOUT THE PROGRAM

This program is open to New Mexico residents who are willing to make a commitment to stay and practice medicine in New Mexico after medical school with a special focus on medically underserved areas and populations. Factors considered for admission include academic excellence, community involvement and volunteer service, a commitment to practice in New Mexico, honors and awards, extracurricular activities, letters of recommendation, personal statement, and medically related experience where available. All students meeting the minimum test scores will be interviewed for the program.

Students in the program are not allowed to apply to any other medical school.

TRANSFER STUDENTS CONSIDERED

No

CITIZENSHIP REQUIREMENTS

New Mexico residents who are current New Mexico high school seniors and high school seniors outside of New Mexico who are enrolled members of the Navajo Tribe and live in the Navajo Nation.

MINIMUM REQUIRED FACTORS IN SELECTION

CLASSES

No specific requirement

GPA

No specific requirement. Average GPA of enrolled students is 4.05.

SAT

Math 510; verbal 450; average SAT of enrolled students is 1,305.

ACT

Math 22; reading 19; science 19; English 19. Average ACT of enrolled students is 31.

ACCEPTANCES

28 students are accepted each year.

FACTORS REQUIRED TO CONTINUE IN PROGRAM

Minimum GPA of 3.37. GPA for pre-med courses must be 3.0.

MCAT REQUIRED

Yes; students must achieve the minimum MCAT score accepted by the school of medicine, generally about a 22; part of the program is a prep class to help students prepare for the MCAT

FINANCIAL AID

All BA/MD undergraduate students are required to apply for all available scholarships. Scholarships received will be deducted from the cost of attending and a grant will be given for the difference for all undergraduates.

COST

	Resident Tuition and Fees ($)	Non Resident Tuition and Fees ($)
Undergraduate	0	not applicable
Medical school	19,395	not applicable

COLLEGE

Hofstra University

MEDICAL SCHOOL

Hofstra North Shore-LIJ School of Medicine

ADDRESS

Undergraduate Admissions
Hofstra University
Hempstead, New York 11549-1000
516-463-6700
www.hofstra.edu/Admission/adm_4plus4.html
bsmd@hofstra.edu

NAME OF PROGRAM

4+4 BS-BA/MD Program

LENGTH OF PROGRAM

8 years

APPLICATION DEADLINE

November 15 or December 15. All supplemental application materials must be received by February1.

INFORMATION ABOUT THE PROGRAM

Students apply to the undergraduate college, and qualified applicants will be requested to submit a supplemental application to the program. The supplemental application will be sent in January. Students may major in any subject.

TRANSFER STUDENTS CONSIDERED

No

CITIZENSHIP REQUIREMENTS

U.S. citizen or permanent resident visa

MINIMUM REQUIRED FACTORS IN SELECTION

CLASSES

Four years of math (with calculus), four years of English, and three years of science (including chemistry and physics)

GPA

Unweighted GPA of 3.7; top ten percent of high school class if the school ranks

SAT

1,350 critical reading and math

ACT

32

ACCEPTANCES

In recent year they have received over 200 application for around 15 spots.

FACTORS REQUIRED TO CONTINUE IN PROGRAM

3.6 undergraduate and science GPA; no course repeated and no grade lower than a B in a science course and no grade lower than a C in a non-science course.

MCAT REQUIRED

Yes; a minimum score on the new MCAT will be determined that will not be greater than the mean score of the previous year's entering class.

FINANCIAL AID

Available for undergraduate students

COST

	Resident Tuition and Fees ($)	Non Resident Tuition and Fees ($)
Undergraduate	39,400	39,400
Medical school	47,000	47,000

COLLEGE

Rensselaer Polytechnic Institute

MEDICAL SCHOOL

Albany Medical College

ADDRESS

Dean of Undergraduate Admissions
Rensselaer Polytechnic Institute
110 Eighth Street
Troy, New York 12180-3590
518-276-6216
http://science.rpi.edu/physician-scientist-program
admissions@rpi.edu

NAME OF PROGRAM

Accelerated Physician-Scientist Program

LENGTH OF PROGRAM

7 years

APPLICATION DEADLINE

November 1

INFORMATION ABOUT THE PROGRAM

The focus of this program is on training physicians in medical research. Students begin research activities in the spring of their junior year at Rensselaer and continue through the summer following the first year at Albany Medical College. This involves about eight months in the laboratory. Students also take a course in the principles of research. Students major in biology.

Rensselaer identifies top students for the program and forwards those applications to Albany Medical College. Albany selects students for interviews; and interviews are conducted in January, February and March. Admissions decisions are made in April.

Motivation to study medicine and maturity are particularly important for admission to this program.

TRANSFER STUDENTS CONSIDERED

No

CITIZENSHIP REQUIREMENTS

U.S. citizen or permanent resident visa

MINIMUM REQUIRED FACTORS IN SELECTION

CLASSES

A year each of biology, chemistry, and physics; four years of math through at least pre-calculus; four years English; and two years of social studies or history.

GPA

No specific requirement

SAT

Most students invited to interview scored a minimum of 1,425 critical reading and math; average score of enrolled students is 1,471. One math subject test and one subject test in biology, chemistry, or physics are required.

ACT

Accepted as alternative to SAT

ACCEPTANCES

Typically receive over 500 applicants for approximately 13 spots

FACTORS REQUIRED TO CONTINUE IN PROGRAM

Minimum 3.5 GPA overall and in science courses. No grade below C.

MCAT REQUIRED

No

FINANCIAL AID

Available for undergraduate students

COST

	Resident Tuition and Fees ($)	Non Resident Tuition and Fees ($)
Undergraduate	48,100	48,100
Medical school	56,614	56,614

COLLEGE
Siena College

MEDICAL SCHOOL
Albany Medical College

ADDRESS
Office of Admissions
Siena College
515 Loudon Road
Loudonville, New York 12211-1462
518-783-2423
www.siena.edu/academics/academics-at-siena
/additional-academic-opportunities
/albany-medical-college-program/
afalvey@siena.edu

NAME OF PROGRAM
Science, Humanities and Medicine Program

LENGTH OF PROGRAM
8 years

APPLICATION DEADLINE
November 15

INFORMATION ABOUT THE PROGRAM
This program places emphasis on humanities, ethics, and community service to the medically underserved. In addition to the
traditional science courses, students take courses in philosophy,
ethics, metaphysics, medical sociology, and healthcare communi-
cations. In the summer after the third year of college, students
engage in nonmedical work with the disadvantaged around the
world. Students graduate with a biology degree and a minor in the
humanities.

Following the second year of medical school, students work in
rural and inner city clinics.

Beyond academics, the admissions committee focuses on leadership, communication skills, and a commitment to service. The
volunteer activities should include some health-related experience.

TRANSFER STUDENTS CONSIDERED
No

CITIZENSHIP REQUIREMENTS
U.S. citizen or permanent resident visa

MINIMUM REQUIRED FACTORS IN SELECTION

CLASSES

Four years of science including biology, chemistry, and physics. Four years of math through at least pre-calculus, with calculus preferred.

GPA

Top ten percent of class

SAT

1,950 with a minimum of 1,300 in critical reading and math. Average score of 640 on SAT critical reading and 730 on SAT math section.

ACT

30

ACCEPTANCES

12–14 new students are selected each year from over 450 applicants.

FACTORS REQUIRED TO CONTINUE IN PROGRAM

3.5 GPA

MCAT REQUIRED

No

FINANCIAL AID

Available for undergraduate students

COST

	Resident Tuition and Fees ($)	Non Resident Tuition and Fees ($)
Undergraduate	33,415	33,415
Medical school	56,614	56,614

COLLEGE
Union College

MEDICAL SCHOOL
Albany Medical College

ADDRESS
Union College
807 Union Street
Schenectady, New York 12308-3103
518-388-6112
www.union.edu/offices/lim/
castillv@union.edu

NAME OF PROGRAM
Leadership in Medicine

LENGTH OF PROGRAM
8 years

APPLICATION DEADLINE
November 15

INFORMATION ABOUT THE PROGRAM
This program is unusual in that it includes a master's degree in addition to the BS and MD degrees. The first four years are spent at Union College, where students complete a biology or chemistry major as well as a second interdepartmental major in the humanities or social sciences. Ten courses in health care management are also included as part of the undergraduate education. The undergraduate program includes two summer sessions in addition to the four years at Union. A term abroad or international experience is also expected during the college years. Students are also involved in a bioethics program and a health services practicum.

A master's degree in science or an MBA is also completed during the four years at Union College. According to the program, they prepare "physicians who will be leaders capable of addressing the managerial, moral, multicultural, and international challenges facing American medicine in the twenty-first century." The focus of the program is on three areas that future leaders in medicine must be familiar with: the economic issues facing medicine, the changing face of biomedical ethics, and the need to maintain a global perspective.

Union identifies top students for the program and forwards those applications to Albany Medical College. Albany selects students for interviews; and interviews are conducted in January, February, and March. Admissions decisions are made in April.

Of particular importance are the personal qualities of motivation, maturity, and personal development.

TRANSFER STUDENTS CONSIDERED

No

CITIZENSHIP REQUIREMENTS

U.S. citizen or permanent resident visa

MINIMUM REQUIRED FACTORS IN SELECTION

CLASSES

Biology and chemistry required; physics preferred

GPA

Top ten percent of high school class

SAT

2,010 minimum SAT; one science and one math subject test, with minimum score of 650 on each test; average SAT scores for new students was 740 critical reading, 724 math, and 748 writing.

ACT

30

ACCEPTANCES

Approximately 80 students are interviewed, and about 40 students enter the program each year.

FACTORS REQUIRED TO CONTINUE IN PROGRAM

3.5 GPA

MCAT REQUIRED

No

FINANCIAL AID

Union College has need-based and merit-based financial aid

COST

	Resident Comprehensive Fee ($)	Non Resident Comprehensive Fee ($)
Undergraduate	62,274	62,274
Medical school	56,614	56,614

COLLEGE

Brooklyn College

MEDICAL SCHOOL

The State University of New York (SUNY) Health Science Center at Brooklyn

ADDRESS

Director, B.A.-M.D. Program
22231 Boylan Hall, Brooklyn College
2900 Bedford Avenue
Brooklyn, New York 11210-2889
718-951-4706
www.brooklyn.cuny.edu/web/academics/honors/academy
/programs/ba-md.php
adminqry@brooklyn.cuny.edu

NAME OF PROGRAM

B.A.-M.D. Program

LENGTH OF PROGRAM

8 years

APPLICATION DEADLINE

December 15

INFORMATION ABOUT THE PROGRAM

Students in the program may major in any field. Students must complete a clinical internship of 320 hours during any summer except the summer following senior year; 60 hours of non-clinical community service is required each semester after freshman year.

TRANSFER STUDENTS CONSIDERED

No

CITIZENSHIP REQUIREMENTS

U.S. citizen or permanent resident visa; must be a resident of New York, New Jersey, or Connecticut, with preference given to New York State residents

MINIMUM REQUIRED FACTORS IN SELECTION

CLASSES

No specific requirement

GPA

Academic average of 90

SAT

1,200 critical reading and math; typical scores of accepted students are between 1,300 and 1,450 on critical reading and math.

ACT

No specific requirement

ACCEPTANCES

There are typically 250–300 applicants. Approximately 100 students are interviewed for 15 spots.

FACTORS REQUIRED TO CONTINUE IN PROGRAM

3.5 overall and science GPA each semester after freshman year

MCAT REQUIRED

Yes; minimum requirements are to be set by the College of Medicine.

FINANCIAL AID

All students admitted to the program are provided a $4,000 a year scholarship.

COST

	Resident Tuition and Fees ($)	Non Resident Tuition and Fees ($)
Undergraduate	6,330	16,800
Medical school	38,250	63,260

COLLEGE
Stony Brook University

MEDICAL SCHOOL
Stony Brook University School of Medicine

ADDRESS
Undergraduate Admissions, Honors Programs
118 Administration Building
Stony Brook University
Stony Brook, New York 11794-1901
631-632-6868
http://mobile.cc.stonybrook.edu/sb/undergraduate-admissions/
academics/honors/#view-medicine-scholars
enroll@stonybrook.edu

NAME OF PROGRAM
Scholars for Medicine Program

LENGTH OF PROGRAM
8 years

APPLICATION DEADLINE
January 15. Additional application materials are due February 1.

INFORMATION ABOUT THE PROGRAM
Students may enter this program from one of two tracks. These
include the Scholars for Medicine Track for select students in
the Honors College and the Women in Science and Engineering
(WISE) or the Engineering Scholars for Medicine track. Students
may only apply to one of these programs. No specific majors are
required. The program provides a series of seminars related to
health-related fields and students may also engage in research.

TRANSFER STUDENTS CONSIDERED
No

CITIZENSHIP REQUIREMENTS
U.S. citizen or permanent resident visa

MINIMUM REQUIRED FACTORS IN SELECTION

CLASSES

No specific requirement

GPA

Ninety-five percent or 3.8 unweighted

SAT

1,350 critical reading and math

ACT

Not accepted

ACCEPTANCES

In recent years approximately 5 students have entered the program each year from over 800 applicants.

FACTORS REQUIRED TO CONTINUE IN PROGRAM

3.4 cumulative GPA and 3.2 science GPA; students in the College of Engineering need a minimum cumulative and science GPA of 3.2.

MCAT REQUIRED

Yes, must score at or above the national average for that test year

FINANCIAL AID

No special financial aid for students in the program

COST

	Resident Tuition and Fees ($)	Non Resident Tuition and Fees ($)
Undergraduate	8,854	23,935
Medical school	44,244	69,254

COLLEGE

Clarkson University

MEDICAL SCHOOL

SUNY Upstate Medical University

ADDRESS

Pre-Health Sciences Advisor
Room 210 Science Center
PO Box 5805
Potsdam, New York 13699-5805
315-268-2391
www.clarkson.edu/admission/upstate_medical/
www.upstate.edu/com/admissions/options/clarkson.php
admission@clarkson.edu

NAME OF PROGRAM

Early Admission Program

LENGTH OF PROGRAM

8 years

APPLICATION DEADLINE

February 1

INFORMATION ABOUT THE PROGRAM

Preference is given to students from an underrepresented minority. Student need to provide a recommendation letter from someone who can describe the student's potential for a career in medicine.

Students must complete 40 hours of community service in a medical setting during their time at Clarkson.

TRANSFER STUDENTS CONSIDERED

No

CITIZENSHIP REQUIREMENTS

U.S. citizen or permanent resident visa; resident of a rural New York community

MINIMUM REQUIRED FACTORS IN SELECTION

CLASSES

No specific requirement

GPA

Ninety percent average

SAT

1,250 critical reading and math

ACT

28

ACCEPTANCES

No information provided

FACTORS REQUIRED TO CONTINUE IN PROGRAM

3.5 overall and science GPA

MCAT REQUIRED

Yes; minimum score of 30 on the old MCAT

FINANCIAL AID

No special financial aid for students in the program

COST

	Resident Tuition and Fees ($)	Non Resident Tuition and Fees ($)
Undergraduate	44,630	not applicable
Medical school	38,250	not applicable

COLLEGE

Hobart and William Smith Colleges

MEDICAL SCHOOL

SUNY Upstate Medical University

ADDRESS

Pre-Health Advisor
Elizabeth Blackwell Medical Scholars Program
Hobart and William Smith Colleges
Office of Admissions, 629 South Main Street
Geneva, New York 14456-3165
800-852-2256
www.upstate.edu/com/admissions/options/blackwell.php
admissions@hws.edu

NAME OF PROGRAM

Elizabeth Blackwell Medical Scholars Program

LENGTH OF PROGRAM

8 years

APPLICATION DEADLINE

January 15

INFORMATION ABOUT THE PROGRAM

To qualify for the program students must meet at least one of
the following criteria: be from a rural background; be from an
underrepresented minority; be the first generation to attend college. During the undergraduate years, students must complete an
internship/shadowing program at related hospitals and complete
enrichment opportunities offered by the medical school. Students
must complete an admissions interview before February 1.

TRANSFER STUDENTS CONSIDERED

No

CITIZENSHIP REQUIREMENTS

U.S. citizen or permanent resident visa

MINIMUM REQUIRED FACTORS IN SELECTION

CLASSES

No specific requirement

GPA

3.7 unweighted or 90 on 100 scale

SAT

1,250 critical reading and math

ACT

28

ACCEPTANCES

No information provided

FACTORS REQUIRED TO CONTINUE IN PROGRAM

3.5 GPA to maintain scholarship eligibility.

MCAT REQUIRED

Yes

FINANCIAL AID

Students accepted into the program receive a $25,000 scholarship for all four years of undergraduate study.

COST

	Resident Tuition and Fees ($)	Non Resident Tuition and Fees ($)
Undergraduate	48,586	48,586
Medical school	38,250	63,260

COLLEGE

St. Bonaventure University

MEDICAL SCHOOL

SUNY Upstate Medical University

ADDRESS

Director Franciscan Health Care Professionals Program
Biology Department
De La Roche Hall, Room 219
St. Bonaventure University
3261 West State Road
St. Bonaventure, New York 14778-9800
716-375-2656
www.sbu.edu/academics/schools/arts-and-sciences
/departments-majors-minors/pre-medicine
/sbu-suny-upstate-dual-admit-program-in-medicine
www.upstate.edu/com/admissions/options/st_bonaventure.php
sbuinfo@sbu.edu

NAME OF PROGRAM

B.S./B.A.–M.D. 4+4 Dual Admission Program

LENGTH OF PROGRAM

8 years

APPLICATION DEADLINE

December 15

INFORMATION ABOUT THE PROGRAM

Preference is given to applicants from rural areas and those with
a strong desire to practice in rural and underserved areas or students from traditionally disadvantaged background. Students being considered with be invited for an interview at St. Bonaventure
in January or February and then invited for an interview at the
medical school in March. A personal statement essay detailing
your interest in the medical field and your interest in St. Bonaventure and Upstate Medical Center is required. A résumé of all of
your extracurricular activities is also required as are two letters
of recommendation including at least one from a science teacher.
Students in the program will participate in the Rural Medical
Scholars Program through SUNY Upstate.

TRANSFER STUDENTS CONSIDERED

No

CITIZENSHIP REQUIREMENTS

U.S. citizen or permanent resident visa; New York residents receive preference.

MINIMUM REQUIRED FACTORS IN SELECTION

CLASSES

No specific requirement

GPA

90 on 100 scale

SAT

1,300 critical reading and math

ACT

29

ACCEPTANCES

Up to 3 students are selected each year

FACTORS REQUIRED TO CONTINUE IN PROGRAM

3.5 minimum GPA overall and in science courses; no grade lower than C

MCAT REQUIRED

Yes; minimum score of 507

FINANCIAL AID

No special financial aid for students in the program.

COST

	Resident Tuition and Fees ($)	Non Resident Tuition and Fees ($)
Undergraduate	31,389	31,389
Medical school	38,250	not applicable

COLLEGE

St. Lawrence University

MEDICAL SCHOOL

SUNY Upstate Medical University

ADDRESS

Director of Admissions
St. Lawrence University
23 Romoda Drive
Canton, New York 13617-1423
800-285-1856
www.stlawu.edu/admissions/rural-medicine-program
www.upstate.edu/com/admissions/options/st_lawrence.php
jfreeman@stlawu.edu

NAME OF PROGRAM

Rural Medicine Program

LENGTH OF PROGRAM

8 years

APPLICATION DEADLINE

December 1

INFORMATION ABOUT THE PROGRAM

Strong preference is given to applicants from a rural setting who
are also first generation college students or from a disadvantaged
economic background. Strong preference is also given to those
students who have a desire to return to practice medicine in an
underserved rural area. Volunteer service and doctor shadowing
during the undergraduate years are also required.

Students complete an application to the college and a separate
application to the program.

TRANSFER STUDENTS CONSIDERED

No

CITIZENSHIP REQUIREMENTS

U.S. citizen or permanent resident visa; preference given to residents of rural New York

MINIMUM REQUIRED FACTORS IN SELECTION

CLASSES
No specific requirement

GPA
Ninety percent average

SAT
1,250 critical reading and math

ACT
27

ACCEPTANCES
No information provided

FACTORS REQUIRED TO CONTINUE IN PROGRAM
Overall and science GPA of 3.5

MCAT REQUIRED
Yes, minimum score of 30 on the old MCAT

FINANCIAL AID
No special financial aid for students in the program.

COST

	Resident Tuition and Fees ($)	Non Resident Tuition and Fees ($)
Undergraduate	49,060	49,060
Medical school	38,250	63,260

COLLEGE
SUNY College of Environmental Science and Forestry

MEDICAL SCHOOL
SUNY Upstate Medical University

ADDRESS
SUNY-ESF
1 Forestry Drive
Syracuse, New York 13210-2712
315-470-6600
www.esf.edu/prehealth/umu.htm
www.upstate.edu/com/admissions/options/suny_esf.php
esfinfo@esf.edu

NAME OF PROGRAM
Joint BS/MD Program

LENGTH OF PROGRAM
8 years

APPLICATION DEADLINE
January 1

INFORMATION ABOUT THE PROGRAM
This program addresses the shortage of physicians in rural New York. The program also is trying to provide a more diverse student population for entry into medical school. Applicants who are considered economically or educationally disadvantaged are given preference. Students in the program will participate in the Rural Medical Scholars Program. Students may major in any program.

TRANSFER STUDENTS CONSIDERED
No

CITIZENSHIP REQUIREMENTS
U.S. citizen or permanent resident visa; New York state residency. Preference given to students from a rural county.

MINIMUM REQUIRED FACTORS IN SELECTION

CLASSES
Four years of science and math

GPA
90 out of 100 GPA

SAT
1,250 critical reading and math

ACT
28

ACCEPTANCES
No information provided

FACTORS REQUIRED TO CONTINUE IN PROGRAM
Overall and science GPA of 3.5

MCAT REQUIRED
Yes; minimum score of 30

FINANCIAL AID
No special financial aid for students in the program

COST

	Resident Tuition and Fees ($)	Non Resident Tuition and Fees ($)
Undergraduate	7,770	not applicable
Medical school	38,250	not applicable

COLLEGE
SUNY Fredonia

MEDICAL SCHOOL
SUNY Upstate Medical University

ADDRESS
SUNY at Fredonia
280 Central Avenue
Fredonia, New York 14063
716-673-3111
www.fredonia.edu/department/biology/prehealth/upstateEAP.asp
Pre-Medicine.Program@fredonia.edu

NAME OF PROGRAM
Joint BS/MD Program

LENGTH OF PROGRAM
8 years

APPLICATION DEADLINE
January 1

INFORMATION ABOUT THE PROGRAM
This program addresses the shortage of physicians in rural New York. The program also is trying to provide a more diverse student population for entry into medical school. Applicants who are considered economically or educationally disadvantaged are given preference. Students in the program will participate in the Rural Medical Scholars Program. Students may major in any program.

TRANSFER STUDENTS CONSIDERED
No

CITIZENSHIP REQUIREMENTS
U.S. citizen or permanent resident visa; New York state residency; preference given to students from a rural county

MINIMUM REQUIRED FACTORS IN SELECTION

CLASSES
Four years of science and math

GPA
Ninety percent average

SAT
1,250 critical reading and math

ACT
28

ACCEPTANCES
No information provided

FAFACTORS REQUIRED TO CONTINUE IN PROGRAM
3.5 overall and science GPA

MCAT REQUIRED
Yes; minimum score of 30

FINANCIAL AID
No special financial aid for students in the program

COST

	Resident Tuition and Fees ($)	Non Resident Tuition and Fees ($)
Undergraduate	8,074	not applicable
Medical school	38,250	not applicable

COLLEGE

SUNY Geneseo

MEDICAL SCHOOL

SUNY Upstate Medical University

ADDRESS

Director of Admissions
SUNY Geneseo
1 College Circle
Geneseo, New York 14454-1401
585-245-5000
www.geneseo.edu/admissions/bsmd-suny-upstate
www.upstate.edu/com/admissions/options/geneseo.php
odonnell@geneseo.edu

NAME OF PROGRAM

BS/MD Early Admittance Program

LENGTH OF PROGRAM

8 years

APPLICATION DEADLINE

January 1

INFORMATION ABOUT THE PROGRAM

Preference given to students who are from a rural community in
New York State and who come from a disadvantaged background.
However, students from more urban backgrounds are also considered. The program is geared to students who wish to practice
family medicine in rural communities after graduation. Students
applying to the program should select biology as your major and
notify the admissions office of your interest in the program. There
is also a required essay detailing your interest and experience in
the health field and your interest in the program through Geneseo. This essay may be emailed to the admissions office.

There are various experiences provided to help support students before attending medical school. Students accepted into the
program will participate in the Rural Medical Scholars Program.

TRANSFER STUDENTS CONSIDERED

No

CITIZENSHIP REQUIREMENTS

U.S. citizen or permanent resident visa; New York resident

MINIMUM REQUIRED FACTORS IN SELECTION

CLASSES
No specific requirement

GPA
Ninety percent average

SAT
1,250 critical reading and math

ACT
28

ACCEPTANCES
No information provided

FACTORS REQUIRED TO CONTINUE IN PROGRAM
3.5 overall and science GPA

MCAT REQUIRED
Yes; minimum score of 30

FINANCIAL AID
No special financial aid for students in the program

COST

	Resident Tuition and Fees ($)	Non Resident Tuition and Fees ($)
Undergraduate	8,113	not applicable
Medical school	38,250	not applicable

COLLEGE
SUNY Potsdam

MEDICAL SCHOOL
SUNY Upstate Medical University

ADDRESS
Director of Admissions
State University of New York at Potsdam
44 Pierrepont Avenue
Potsdam, New York 13676-2200
315-267-2000
www.upstate.edu/com/admissions/options/potsdam.php
nesbittw@potsdam.edu

NAME OF PROGRAM
Special Admissions Options

LENGTH OF PROGRAM
8 years

APPLICATION DEADLINE
No information provided

INFORMATION ABOUT THE PROGRAM
Preference given to students who come from a rural area of New York State and come from a disadvantaged background. Students accepted into the program will participate in the Rural Medical Scholars Program.

TRANSFER STUDENTS CONSIDERED
No

CITIZENSHIP REQUIREMENTS
U.S. citizen or permanent resident visa, New York State residents

MINIMUM REQUIRED FACTORS IN SELECTION

CLASSES

No specific requirements

GPA

90 out of 100

SAT

1,250 critical reading and math

ACT

28

ACCEPTANCES

No information provided

FACTORS REQUIRED TO CONTINUE IN PROGRAM

Overall and science GPA of 3.5

MCAT REQUIRED

Yes; minimum score of 30

FINANCIAL AID

No special financial aid for students in the program

COST

	Resident Tuition and Fees ($)	Non Resident Tuition and Fees ($)
Undergraduate	7,885	not applicable
Medical school	38,250	not applicable

COLLEGE
Wilkes University

MEDICAL SCHOOL
SUNY Upstate Medical University

ADDRESS
Wilkes University
84 West South Street
Wilkes-Barre, Pennsylvanian 18766-0003
800-945-5378
www.upstate.edu/com/admissions/options/guthrie.php
Sharp@wilkes.edu

NAME OF PROGRAM
Guthrie Pre-Medical Scholars Program

LENGTH OF PROGRAM
8 years

APPLICATION DEADLINE
November 15

INFORMATION ABOUT THE PROGRAM
The purpose of this program is to increase the number of physicians interested in serving in rural health care delivery systems. This program requires three interviews including one at Wilkes, one at a local clinical site, and one at the SUNY Upstate medical school. Students accepted into the program will participate in the Rural Medical Scholars Program and study rural health care by pursuing clinical coursework and research at the Guthrie-Robert Packer Medical Center.

TRANSFER STUDENTS CONSIDERED
No

CITIZENSHIP REQUIREMENTS
U.S. citizen or permanent resident visa; must reside in a rural county in the Southern Tier of New York State

MINIMUM REQUIRED FACTORS IN SELECTION

CLASSES

Four years of math, English, science, and social studies

GPA

Top ten percent of high school class

SAT

1,200 critical reading and math

ACT

27

ACCEPTANCES

No information provided

FACTORS REQUIRED TO CONTINUE IN PROGRAM

3.5 overall and science GPA

MCAT REQUIRED

Yes; minimum score of 30

FINANCIAL AID

No special financial aid for students in the program

COST

	Resident Tuition and Fees ($)	Non Resident Tuition and Fees ($)
Undergraduate	32,356	not applicable
Medical school	38,250	not applicable

COLLEGE

University of Rochester

MEDICAL SCHOOL

University of Rochester School of Medicine

ADDRESS

Office of Admissions
PO Box 270251
Rochester, New York 14627-0251
585-275-3221
http://enrollment.rochester.edu/professional/REMS/
admit@admissions.rochester.edu

NAME OF PROGRAM

Rochester Early Medical Scholars (REMS)

LENGTH OF PROGRAM

8 years

APPLICATION DEADLINE

December 1

INFORMATION ABOUT THE PROGRAM

Students in the REMS program may major in any subject and are encouraged to explore all of the academic offerings of the university. The most popular majors are biology, chemistry, and health and society. Students are required to complete a social service project before enrolling in the medical school. REMS students may also apply to any of the other combined degree programs available at the University including MD/PhD, MD/MPH, MD/MBA and MD/MS programs.

The school of medicine's Double-Helix curriculum integrates the basic science and clinical science aspects of medical school across all four years of the medical school experience. This means that the medical students begin clinical clerkships in January of the first year. The medical school encourages critical thinking, problem solving, and active learning in small groups.

Summer research programs and international experiences are available for REMS undergraduates and medical students.

Advantages of the REMS program include faculty mentors; seminars; support and social events; academic freedom; problem-based learning; and funding for summer research.

TRANSFER STUDENTS CONSIDERED

No

CITIZENSHIP REQUIREMENTS

International students considered for program

MINIMUM REQUIRED FACTORS IN SELECTION

CLASSES

No specific requirement

GPA

No minimum but the strongest applicants have a 3.95 unweighted GPA with strong college prep courses and top three percent of their high school class.

SAT

No minimum but strongest applicants have at least a 1,450 SAT score on the critical reading and math and at least 700 on SAT writing. Average SAT critical reading score is 716, average SAT math score is 726, and average writing score is 728.

SAT SUBJECT TESTS

No minimum and not required. However, applicants are strongly encouraged to take a subject test in biology or chemistry and a subject test in math level 1 or math level 2. Strongest applicants score 700 or above on each of these subject tests.

ACT

No minimum but strongest applicants have at least a 34.

ACCEPTANCES

In past years, approximately 15 students have been accepted from over 400 applications.

FACTORS REQUIRED TO CONTINUE IN PROGRAM

Students must have an overall GPA of 3.3 and a math and science GPA of 3.3 after freshman year, a 3.4 GPA overall and in math and science courses after sophomore year, and a 3.5 overall GPA and math and science GPA after junior year in college.

MCAT REQUIRED

No

FINANCIAL AID

The University of Rochester meets one hundred percent of the demonstrated need for a student's undergraduate education.

COST

	Resident Tuition and Fees ($)	Non Resident Tuition and Fees ($)
Undergraduate	48,290	48,290
Medical school	52,799	52,799

COLLEGE
East Carolina University

MEDICAL SCHOOL
East Carolina University Brody School of Medicine

ADDRESS
Office of Admissions
East Carolina University
600 Moye Boulevard
Greenville, North Carolina 27834-4300
252-328-6373
www.ecu.edu/bsomadmissions/assurance.cfm
somadmissions@ecu.edu

NAME OF PROGRAM
Early Assurance Program

LENGTH OF PROGRAM
8 years

APPLICATION DEADLINE
November 15

INFORMATION ABOUT THE PROGRAM
Students must be admitted to the Honors College to be considered
for the program. There are numerous group and enrichment activities for students in the program, including hands-on medical
exposure, summer programs, and service learning.

TRANSFER STUDENTS CONSIDERED
No

CITIZENSHIP REQUIREMENTS
U.S. citizen or permanent resident visa; North Carolina residents
only

MINIMUM REQUIRED FACTORS IN SELECTION

CLASSES
No specific requirement

GPA
3.5 unweighted or 4.0 weighted

SAT
1,200 (superscoring allowed)

ACT
27 (superscoring allowed)

ACCEPTANCES
4 spots available per year

FACTORS REQUIRED TO CONTINUE IN PROGRAM
3.5 overall and science GPA

MCAT REQUIRED
No

FINANCIAL AID
No special financial aid for students in the program

COST

	Resident Tuition and Fees ($)	Non Resident Tuition and Fees ($)
Undergraduate	6,580	not applicable
Medical school	20,558	not applicable

COLLEGE
North Carolina A&T State University

MEDICAL SCHOOL
East Carolina University Brody School of Medicine

ADDRESS
North Carolina A&T State University
1601 North Market Street
Greensboro, North Carolina 27411
336-334-7500
http://ncatearlyassurance.yolasite.com/
cdwhite@ncat.edu

NAME OF PROGRAM
Early Assurance Scholars Program

LENGTH OF PROGRAM
8 years

APPLICATION DEADLINE
February 1

INFORMATION ABOUT THE PROGRAM
Students applying to the program must complete a program-specific application. Only the top two students selected have guaranteed admittance to the Brody School of Medicine. These two students will not need to take the MCAT if their SAT critical reading and math are greater than 1,200. The remaining students will follow a common curriculum and be prepared to take the MCAT at the end of the junior year if necessary.

TRANSFER STUDENTS CONSIDERED
No

CITIZENSHIP REQUIREMENTS
U.S. citizen or permanent resident visa; North Carolina residents only

MINIMUM REQUIRED FACTORS IN SELECTION

CLASSES

No specific requirement

GPA

No specific requirement

SAT

1,200. Students with SAT critical reading and math scores between 1,000 and 1,199 will be required to take the MCAT.

ACT

No specific requirement

ACCEPTANCES

Eight students will be selected to participate in the program. The top two students will be guaranteed admission to the medical school.

FACTORS REQUIRED TO CONTINUE IN PROGRAM

3.5 overall GPA

MCAT REQUIRED

Yes, for some students. If they are required to take the MCAT they must score at least an 8 on each section of the MCAT.

FINANCIAL AID

No special financial aid for students in the program

COST

	Resident Tuition and Fees ($)	Non Resident Tuition and Fees ($)
Undergraduate	7,700	not applicable
Medical school	20,558	not applicable

COLLEGE
Case Western Reserve University

MEDICAL SCHOOL
Case Western Reserve University School of Medicine

ADDRESS
Office of Undergraduate Admission
Wolstein Hall, Case Western Reserve University
10900 Euclid Avenue
Cleveland, Ohio 44106-7055
216-368-4450
http://admission.case.edu/academics/ppsp.aspx
admission@case.edu

NAME OF PROGRAM
Pre-Professional Scholars Program

LENGTH OF PROGRAM
8 years

APPLICATION DEADLINE
December 1

INFORMATION ABOUT THE PROGRAM
Students who complete the undergraduate program in less than four years may not enter the medical school early and are required to spend any available time involved in experiences that will enhance their personal or professional development. No specific majors are required, although the most common are biology and biochemistry.

TRANSFER STUDENTS CONSIDERED
No

CITIZENSHIP REQUIREMENTS
International students considered

MINIMUM REQUIRED FACTORS IN SELECTION

CLASSES

One year each of biology, chemistry, and physics as well as four years of math

GPA

No minimum, although typical candidates are in the top ten percent of their high school class

SAT

No minimum, although typical candidates score between 2,200 and 2,300 on SAT; for recent entering class, scores ranged from 710 to 800 on critical reading, 710 to 800 on math, and 710 to 800 on writing

ACT

No minimum, although typical candidates score between 31 and 34

ACCEPTANCES

25–30 students are admitted each year.

FACTORS REQUIRED TO CONTINUE IN PROGRAM

B+ level of performance in college coursework

MCAT REQUIRED

No; students who choose to take it must score 33 or above on the old MCAT; MCAT is required for some scholarship programs.

FINANCIAL AID

No special financial aid for students in the program

COST

	Resident Tuition and Fees ($)	Non Resident Tuition and Fees ($)
Undergraduate	44,156	44,156
Medical school	57,475	57,475

COLLEGE

Kent State University; University of Akron;
Youngstown State University

MEDICAL SCHOOL

Northeast Ohio Medical University

ADDRESS

Office of Admissions
Northeast Ohio Medical University
4209 State Route 44
PO Box 95
Rootstown, Ohio 44272-0095
330-325-6270
www.neomed.edu/admissions/medicine/bsmd
admission@neomed.edu

NAME OF PROGRAM

B.S./M.D. Program

LENGTH OF PROGRAM

6 or 7 years

APPLICATION DEADLINE

November 16

INFORMATION ABOUT THE PROGRAM

Unlike most other programs, the student applies to the medical
school directly and, if chosen, is assigned a college for the first two
to three years of the program. Strong preference is given to Ohio
residents and in particular those students who are interested in
primary medicine in the Northeast Ohio area. Students have the
option of completing the undergraduate portion of the program
in two or three years, where students attend classes year round.
During their undergraduate years students will have premedical
involvement through various activities and seminars. The program will not consider any materials or letters of recommendation
beyond what they specifically request.

TRANSFER STUDENTS CONSIDERED

No

CITIZENSHIP REQUIREMENTS

U.S. citizen or permanent resident visa; preference given to Ohio
residents

MINIMUM REQUIRED FACTORS IN SELECTION

CLASSES

Four years of math, science (including biology, chamistry, and physics), English, social studies, and a foreign language are recommended.

GPA

3.5; accepted student average 3.88; 25th to 75th percentile is 3.81 to 4.00.

SAT

Accepted students average 1,413; 25th to 75th percentile is 1,308 to 1,455 on the critical reading and math sections.

ACT

27; accepted students average 31; 25th to 75th percentile is 29 to 32.

ACCEPTANCES

Each college is given 35 students from the program for a total class of 105. No more than ten percent of the class is from outside Ohio.

FACTORS REQUIRED TO CONTINUE IN PROGRAM

Students must have a 3.2 science and math GPA and a 3.25 over-all GPA and earn at least an 8 on each section of the MCAT to advance to the medical school after two or three years. If you have a 3.5 overall and science and math GPA, you can advance with an MCAT score of 24 with one score of 7. Students are expected to have at least a B in all required math and science courses. Mandatory classes must have a minimum C− grade.

MCAT REQUIRED

Yes; must receive at least an 8 on each section of the test

FINANCIAL AID

There are merit-based scholarships available.

COST

	Resident Tuition and Fees ($)	Non Resident Tuition and Fees ($)
Undergraduate	varies	varies
Medical school	37,943	72,613

COLLEGE
University of Cincinnati

MEDICAL SCHOOL
University of Cincinnati College of Medicine

ADDRESS
University of Cincinnati
231 Albert Sabin Way
Cincinnati, Ohio 45267-2827
513-558-5581
http://med.uc.edu/DualAdmissions.aspx
hs2md@uc.edu

NAME OF PROGRAM
Connections Dual Admissions Program

LENGTH OF PROGRAM
8 years

APPLICATION DEADLINE
November 10

INFORMATION ABOUT THE PROGRAM
Students must also participate as members of the honors program at the university. The program is not binding, and students in the college may apply to other medical schools without penalty. There are various enrichment opportunities available for students in the program. Students must complete both the university undergraduate application as well as the Connection Program application. These are separate applications. Students majoring in biomedical engineering will take 9 years to complete the program.

Students admitted to the program will also be admitted to the Undergraduate Program in Biomedical Sciences and Medicine which provides integrated academic and mentoring opportunities with the College of Medicine.

TRANSFER STUDENTS CONSIDERED
No

CITIZENSHIP REQUIREMENTS
U.S. citizen or permanent resident visa; preference given to Ohio residents

MINIMUM REQUIRED FACTORS IN SELECTION

CLASSES

No specific requirement

GPA

No specific requirement; average unweighted GPA of admitted students is 3.97, and average weighted GPA is 4.60.

SAT

1,300 critical reading and math; average SAT of students admitted to the program is 1,515.

ACT

29; average ACT of students admitted to the program is 34.

ACCEPTANCES

In 2014, 8 students were admitted to the program from 234 applications. Two-thirds of the students were non-Ohio residents.

FACTORS REQUIRED TO CONTINUE IN PROGRAM

3.5 science and overall GPA; graduation from the University Honors Program

MCAT REQUIRED

Yes; a minimum score is required to be determined

FINANCIAL AID

No special financial aid for students in the program

COST

	Resident Tuition and Fees ($)	Non Resident Tuition and Fees ($)
Undergraduate	11,000	26,334
Medical school	29,680	47,944

COLLEGE
University of Oklahoma

MEDICAL SCHOOL
University of Oklahoma College of Medicine

ADDRESS
Program Director
Joe C. and Carol Kerr McClendon Honors College
David L. Boren Hall
1300 Asp Avenue
Norman, Oklahoma 73019-6061
405-325-5291
www.ou.edu/content/honors/specialprograms
/MedHumanitiesScholarship.html
honors@ou.edu

NAME OF PROGRAM
Medical Humanities Scholars Program

LENGTH OF PROGRAM
7 or 8 years

APPLICATION DEADLINE
December 1; January 8

INFORMATION ABOUT THE PROGRAM
Students applying to the program must submit three separate applications. The regular application and the application to the Honors College are available online and are due by December 1. The Medical Humanities Scholars Program application is due in early January. This application is available online, but four copies must be submitted through regular mail.

Students may major in any subject but will self-design a minor in medical humanities. During the undergraduate years students participate in mini internships with both private and academic physicians. Students are encouraged to take a full four years for the undergraduate portion of the program but may petition for approval to obtain their undergraduate degree after three years.

TRANSFER STUDENTS CONSIDERED
No

CITIZENSHIP REQUIREMENTS

U.S. citizen or permanent resident visa; must graduate from a U.S. high school. There is no in-state preference.

MINIMUM REQUIRED FACTORS IN SELECTION

No specific requirement

ACCEPTANCES

They receive 60–70 applications per year and invite approximately 15 students to interview; 5–8 new students enter the program each year.

FACTORS REQUIRED TO CONTINUE IN PROGRAM

Student must have a GPA and MCAT score equal to or higher than the average GPA and MCAT scores of the previous year's entering class.

MCAT REQUIRED

Yes

FINANCIAL AID

No special financial aid for students in the program

COST

	Resident Tuition and Fees ($)	Non Resident Tuition and Fees ($)
Undergraduate	7,102	21,827
Medical school	25,851	55,197

COLLEGE
Drexel University

MEDICAL SCHOOL
Drexel University College of Medicine

ADDRESS
Drexel University Undergraduate Admissions
PO Box 34789
Philadelphia, Pennsylvania 19101-4789
215-895-2000
www.drexel.edu/undergrad/apply/freshmen-instructions
/accelerated/
enroll@drexel.edu

NAME OF PROGRAM
BA/BS/MD

LENGTH OF PROGRAM
7 or 8 years

APPLICATION DEADLINE
November 4

INFORMATION ABOUT THE PROGRAM
Students majoring in the biological sciences, chemistry, psychology or the bachelor of science in engineering can apply to the seven-year program. There is also an eight-year option for students majoring in biomedical engineering or general engineering. Students must submit an application to the undergraduate college as well as a College of Medicine supplemental application. Two letters of recommendation are required; one must be from a high school counselor and the other from a science teacher.

TRANSFER STUDENTS CONSIDERED
No

CITIZENSHIP REQUIREMENTS
U.S. citizen or permanent resident visa; must graduate from a U.S. high school

MINIMUM REQUIRED FACTORS IN SELECTION

CLASSES

Four years of math, English, and lab science, including one year each of biology, chemistry, and physics

GPA

Graduate from U.S. high school in top ten percent of class with 3.5 unweighted GPA; average high school GPA for a recent class was 4.05.

SAT

1,360 critical reading and math; average SAT score for a recent class was 1,538; SAT subject tests are recommended.

ACT

31; average ACT score for a recent class was 34

ACCEPTANCES

In recents years approximately 30 students have been admitted from about 1,000 applications.

FACTORS REQUIRED TO CONTINUE IN PROGRAM

3.5 overall and science GPA with no grade less than C

MCAT REQUIRED

Yes, a minimum score of 506, with minimum of 125 in the psychological, social, and biological foundations of behavior subsection and a minimum of 127 on all other sections, is anticipated.

FINANCIAL AID

No special financial aid for students in the program

COST

	Resident Tuition and Fees ($)	Non Resident Tuition and Fees ($)
Undergraduate	48,756	48,756
Medical school	54,698	54,698

COLLEGE
Lehigh University

MEDICAL SCHOOL
Drexel University College of Medicine

ADDRESS
Office of Admissions
Lehigh University
27 Memorial Drive West
Bethlehem, Pennsylvania 18015-3027
610-758-3100
www.lehigh.edu/bio/UG/UG_Combined.html#medicine
admissions@lehigh.edu

NAME OF PROGRAM
Combined Degree Program in Medicine

LENGTH OF PROGRAM
7 years

APPLICATION DEADLINE
November 15

INFORMATION ABOUT THE PROGRAM
Students may major in any subject at Lehigh, although there are
a number of required courses for the program, so careful planning
is required.

TRANSFER STUDENTS CONSIDERED
No

CITIZENSHIP REQUIREMENTS
U.S. citizen or permanent resident visa

MINIMUM REQUIRED FACTORS IN SELECTION

CLASSES

No specific requirement

GPA

Top five percent of high school class; recently accepted students had an average 3.7 unweighted GPA.

SAT

1,360 critical reading and math; recently accepted students had on average 720 critical reading score and a 780 math score; Subject tests highly recommended—math level 1 or 2 and chemistry.

ACT

31

ACCEPTANCES

In recent years approximately 2 students were admitted from over 200 applications.

FACTORS REQUIRED TO CONTINUE IN PROGRAM

3.5 overall and science and math GPA with no grade less than a C

MCAT REQUIRED

Yes; minimum score on the old MCAT of 9 on verbal section and 10 on each of the science sections; alternatively, a combined score of 31 with no sub-score below 8

FINANCIAL AID

No special financial aid for students in the program

COST

	Resident Tuition and Fees ($)	Non Resident Tuition and Fees ($)
Undergraduate	46,230	46,230
Medical school	54,698	54,698

COLLEGE
Monmouth University

MEDICAL SCHOOL
Drexel University College of Medicine

ADDRESS
Office of Undergraduate Admission
Monmouth University
400 Cedar Avenue
West Long Branch, New Jersey 07764-1898
732-571-3456
www.monmouth.edu/academics/pre-professional_health
/medical_scholars.asp

NAME OF PROGRAM
Monmouth Medical Center Scholars Program

LENGTH OF PROGRAM
8 years

APPLICATION DEADLINE
December 1

INFORMATION ABOUT THE PROGRAM
The focus of this program is on training students who wish to
enter family medicine, internal medicine, or pediatrics. Students
participate in health-related activities at Monmouth Medical Center, including preceptorship in clinical medicine. The program
also provides career counseling, MCAT preparation, and practice interviews. There are two applications for this program, one
to Monmouth University and a Drexel University supplemental
application.

TRANSFER STUDENTS CONSIDERED
No

CITIZENSHIP REQUIREMENTS
U.S. citizen or permanent resident visa; New Jersey residents only

MINIMUM REQUIRED FACTORS IN SELECTION

CLASSES

No specific requirement

GPA

3.5 unweighted

SAT

1,900; 1,270 critical reading and math, with no sub-score lower than 560

ACT

28

ACCEPTANCES

Approximately 8–12 students are invited for the interview process and are narrowed down to 5 selected students each year.

FACTORS REQUIRED TO CONTINUE IN PROGRAM

3.5 overall and science GPA with no grade less than a C in any class

MCAT REQUIRED

Yes; minimum score on the old MCAT of 10 on biological and physical science sections and 9 on verbal section; alternatively, a minimum total score of 31 with no subsection score less than 8.

FINANCIAL AID

No special financial aid for students in the program

COST

	Resident Tuition and Fees ($)	Non Resident Tuition and Fees ($)
Undergraduate	34,128	not applicable
Medical school	54,698	not applicable

COLLEGE

Muhlenberg College

MEDICAL SCHOOL

Drexel University College of Medicine

ADDRESS

Coordinator of 4-4 Program
Office of Admission
Muhlenberg College
2400 Chew Street
Allentown, Pennsylvania 18104-5586
484-664-3200
www.muhlenberg.edu/admissions/cooperativeprogramdrexel4-4/
sconrad@muhlenberg.edu

NAME OF PROGRAM

4-4 Early Assurance Program

LENGTH OF PROGRAM

8 years

APPLICATION DEADLINE

January 1

INFORMATION ABOUT THE PROGRAM

Personal interviews with Muhlenberg are required and must be
completed by the January 1 deadline. Students have the opportunity to participate in research and additional educational enrichment opportunities at Easton Hopital and Drexel during their
undergraduate years.

TRANSFER STUDENTS CONSIDERED

No

CITIZENSHIP REQUIREMENTS

U.S. citizen or permanent resident visa; Canadian residents also
considered. Preference given to students who reside in the Middle
Atlantic Region of Pennsylvania, New Jersey, New York, Dela-
ware or Maryland.

MINIMUM REQUIRED FACTORS IN SELECTION

CLASSES

No specific requirement

GPA

No specific requirements; successful students are normally in the top five percent of their high school class. The average unweighted GPA was 3.65.

SAT

1,270 critical reading and math with no sub-score less than 560; Successful students normally score 1,300 or higher on the critical reading and math.

ACT

29

ACCEPTANCES

This program accepts up to 6 students per year.

FACTORS REQUIRED TO CONTINUE IN PROGRAM

3.5 overall and science GPA

MCAT REQUIRED

Yes. Minimum score on the old MCAT of 10 on the biological and physical science sections and a 9 on the verbal section

FINANCIAL AID

No special financial aid for students in the program

COST

	Resident Tuition and Fees ($)	Non Resident Tuition and Fees ($)
Undergraduate	45,875	45,875
Medical school	54,698	54,698

COLLEGE

Robert Morris University

MEDICAL SCHOOL

Drexel University College of Medicine

ADDRESS

Robert Morris University
6001 University Boulevard
Moon Township, Pennsylvania 15108-2574
800-762-0097
http://rmu.edu/Undergraduate/AcademicOfferings
/Pre-Medicine#Opportunities

NAME OF PROGRAM

Scholars Articulation Program

LENGTH OF PROGRAM

8 years

APPLICATION DEADLINE

No information provided

INFORMATION ABOUT THE PROGRAM

This program is a collaboration between Robert Morris University, Drexel University College of Medicine, and Allegheny General Hospital with the intention of increasing the number of physicians serving Western Pennsylvania. As undergraduates, students participate in a research course and pre-professional internship at Allegheny General Hospital. Preference in admissions is given to students interested in family medicine, general internal medicine, and general pediatrics.

TRANSFER STUDENTS CONSIDERED

No

CITIZENSHIP REQUIREMENTS

U.S. citizen or permanent resident visa; preference given to residents of Ohio, Pennsylvania and West Virginia.

MINIMUM REQUIRED FACTORS IN SELECTION

CLASSES

No specific requirements

GPA

3.5 unweighted

SAT

1,270 critical reading and math

ACT

24

ACCEPTANCES

A maximum of 5 students are accepted each year.

FACTORS REQUIRED TO CONTINUE IN PROGRAM

Overall and science GPA of 3.5

MCAT REQUIRED

Yes; minimum 31

FINANCIAL AID

No special financial aid for students in the program

COST

	Resident Tuition and Fees ($)	Non Resident Tuition and Fees ($)
Undergraduate	25,650	25,650
Medical school	54,698	54,698

COLLEGE
Rosemont College

MEDICAL SCHOOL
Drexel University College of Medicine

ADDRESS
Rosemont College
Office of Admissions
1400 Montgomery Avenue
Rosemont, Pennsylvania 19010-1631
610-526-2966
www.rosemont.edu/academics/undergraduate/special-programs
/collaborative-programs.php
admissions@rosemont.edu

NAME OF PROGRAM
Early Assurance Program/Fast Track Program

LENGTH OF PROGRAM
7 or 8 years

APPLICATION DEADLINE
December 1

INFORMATION ABOUT THE PROGRAM
Rosemont has two programs with Drexel. The Early Assurance Program is an eight-year program. The Fast Track Program is a seven-year program. Students are required to interview at Rosemont as well as Drexel. Students who meet the minimum requirements for the program will receive a Drexel College of Medicine supplemental application, which must be submitted by January 1.

TRANSFER STUDENTS CONSIDERED
No

CITIZENSHIP REQUIREMENTS
U.S. citizen or permanent resident visa

MINIMUM REQUIRED FACTORS IN SELECTION

CLASSES

Full academic course load including three years of foreign language, four years of English and math, as well as at least one semester each of biology, chemistry, and physics.

GPA

Top ten percent of high school class and 3.5 unweighted GPA

SAT

1,300 critical reading and math with no sub-score below 600 for the Early Assurance Program; 1,360 critical reading and math with no sub-score below 560 for the Fast Track Program; writing score is not considered.

ACT

29 for Early Assurance Program; 31 for Fast Track Program

ACCEPTANCES

No information provided

FACTORS REQUIRED TO CONTINUE IN PROGRAM

3.5 GPA and 3.25 science GPA

MCAT REQUIRED

Yes, 506; minimum score of 125 on the Psychological, Social, and Biological Foundations of Behavior section and minimum scores of 127 on all other sections

FINANCIAL AID

No special financial aid for students in the program

COST

	Resident Tuition and Fees ($)	Non Resident Tuition and Fees ($)
Undergraduate	18,000	18,500
Medical school	54,698	54,698

COLLEGE

Ursinus College

MEDICAL SCHOOL

Drexel University College of Medicine

ADDRESS

Ursinus College
Office of Admission
601 E. Main Street
Collegeville, Pennsylvania 19426-1000
610-409-3000
www.ursinus.edu/netcommunity/page.aspx?pid=440
admission@ursinus.edu

NAME OF PROGRAM

Early Assurance Program

LENGTH OF PROGRAM

8 years

APPLICATION DEADLINE

November 1

INFORMATION ABOUT THE PROGRAM

Students must apply in the Early Action 1 deadline, indicating their interest in the Early Assurance Program. Top candidates for the program are chosen in December and then sent additional information about the program. These candidates are interviewed by the undergraduate college in January, and decisions are made on who to recommend to the medical school. The medical school will decide who to interview in February.

TRANSFER STUDENTS CONSIDERED

No

CITIZENSHIP REQUIREMENTS

U.S. citizen or permanent resident visa; must be a graduate of a U.S. high school

MINIMUM REQUIRED FACTORS IN SELECTION

CLASSES

Four years of English and math, three years of science including one year each of biology, chemistry and physics

GPA

Top ten percent of high school class

SAT

1,300 critical reading and math with no sub-score below 560; writing score is not considered.

ACT

No specific requirement

ACCEPTANCES

A maximum of 4 students will be accepted each year.

FACTORS REQUIRED TO CONTINUE IN PROGRAM

3.5 overall and science GPA with no grade less than a C in any class

MCAT REQUIRED

Yes, minimum score on the old MCAT of 10 on biological and physical science sections and 9 on verbal section. Alternatively, a minimum total score of 31 with no subsection score less than 8

FINANCIAL AID

No special financial aid for students in the program

COST

	Resident Tuition and Fees ($)	Non Resident Tuition and Fees ($)
Undergraduate	47,700	47,700
Medical school	54,698	54,698

COLLEGE
Villanova University

MEDICAL SCHOOL
Drexel University College of Medicine

ADDRESS
Health Professions Advisor
Villanova University
800 Lancaster Avenue
Villanova, Pennsylvania 19085-1603
610-519-6000
www1.villanova.edu/villanova/artsci/undergrad
/resources/health/affiliates/medicine.html
hpa@villanova.edu

NAME OF PROGRAM
Medical Affiliate Program

LENGTH OF PROGRAM
7 years

APPLICATION DEADLINE
November 1

INFORMATION ABOUT THE PROGRAM
Students may major in any major offered by Villanova, although
some majors are more difficult to complete in the three years the
student is at the college. The most common major is biology, followed by comprehensive science and biochemistry. Students who
meet the basic requirements will be asked to submit a supplemental application to the medical school.

TRANSFER STUDENTS CONSIDERED
No

CITIZENSHIP REQUIREMENTS
U.S. citizen or permanent resident visa; must be a graduate of a
U.S. high school

MINIMUM REQUIRED FACTORS IN SELECTION

CLASSES

Four years of math, four years of English, three years of science including at least one semester each of biology, chemistry, and physics

GPA

Top five percent of class; 3.8 unweighted; average GPA for admitted students was 3.90 unweighted

SAT

1,380 critical reading and math with no sub-score below 600; SAT subject tests recommended but not required

ACT

31 plus writing

ACCEPTANCES

In recent years this program has accepted approximately 7 students.

FACTORS REQUIRED TO CONTINUE IN PROGRAM

Students must maintain a 3.5 overall and science GPA; no grade less than a C

MCAT REQUIRED

Yes, with minimum score of 506; minimum score of 125 on the Psychological, Social, and Biological Foundations of Behavior sectoin and minimum scores of 127 on all other sections

FINANCIAL AID

No special financial aid for students in the program

COST

	Resident Tuition and Fees ($)	Non Resident Tuition and Fees ($)
Undergraduate	47,266	47,266
Medical school	54,698	54,698

COLLEGE
West Chester University

MEDICAL SCHOOL
Drexel University College of Medicine

ADDRESS
West Chester University of Pennsylvania
700 South High Street
West Chester, Pennsylvania 19383-0001
610-436-1000
www.wcupa.edu/_ACADEMICS/SCH_CAS/MED/Early
_Assurance_Undergrad/drexel.asp
pmed@wcupa.edu

NAME OF PROGRAM
Pre-Medical Program

LENGTH OF PROGRAM
8 years

APPLICATION DEADLINE
November 14

INFORMATION ABOUT THE PROGRAM
Students must submit an application to the college and a supplemental application to Drexel College of Medicine. Students must have documented health care experience.

TRANSFER STUDENTS CONSIDERED
No

CITIZENSHIP REQUIREMENTS
U.S. citizen or permanent resident visa

MINIMUM REQUIRED FACTORS IN SELECTION

CLASSES

Four years of English and math, three years of science including one year each of biology, chemistry and physics

GPA

Top ten percent of high school class and unweighted GPA of 3.5

SAT

1,300 critical reading and math, with no sub-score lower than 560

ACT

No specific requirement

ACCEPTANCES

No information provided

FACTORS REQUIRED TO CONTINUE IN PROGRAM

3.5 overall and science GPA with no grade lower than C in any course

MCAT REQUIRED

Yes, with minimum score on the old MCAT of 9 on verbal reasoning, 10 in physical sciences, and 10 in biological sciences, or a combined score of 31 with no sub-score less than 8

FINANCIAL AID

No special financial aid for students in the program

COST

	Resident Tuition and Fees ($)	Non Resident Tuition and Fees ($)
Undergraduate	9,462	20,280
Medical school	54,698	54,698

COLLEGE
Penn State University

MEDICAL SCHOOL
Jefferson Medical College

ADDRESS
Penn State University
Eberly College of Science
Undergraduate Recruitment Office
108 Whitmore Laboratory
University Park, Pennsylvania 16802-1014
814-865-2609
www.science.psu.edu/premed/premedmed
/accelerated-premed-medical/
admissions@psu.edu

NAME OF PROGRAM
Penn State's Accelerated Premedical-Medical Program

LENGTH OF PROGRAM
7 years

APPLICATION DEADLINE
November 30

INFORMATION ABOUT THE PROGRAM
Note that the six-year option is no longer available. This is a seven-year program only.
Non-academic factors considered include motivation, compassion, integrity, and dedication. Students follow a carefully planned schedule of courses throughout their undergraduate years.

TRANSFER STUDENTS CONSIDERED
No

CITIZENSHIP REQUIREMENTS
International students considered; preference given to qualified residents of Pennsylvania

MINIMUM REQUIRED FACTORS IN SELECTION

CLASSES

Four years of English, three and one half years of math, three years of science, and five years of social studies, humanities, or arts.

GPA

Top ten percent of high school class

SAT

2,100 from a single test date; average test score for class entering 2012 was 2,260

ACT

32 with writing section

ACCEPTANCES

Approximately 25 students start the program each year.

FACTORS REQUIRED TO CONTINUE IN PROGRAM

3.5 overall and science GPA

MCAT REQUIRED

Yes; minimum of 504 with no score less than 126 on any subsection

FINANCIAL AID

Students not eligible for tuition scholarships from Schreyer Honors College or Braddock Scholarships from the Eberly College of Science

COST

	Resident Tuition and Fees ($)	Non Resident Tuition and Fees ($)
Undergraduate	16,572	30,404
Medical school	54,161	54,161

COLLEGE
Wilkes University

MEDICAL SCHOOL
Penn State Hershey College of Medicine

ADDRESS
Wilkes University
84 West South Street
Wilkes-Barre, Pennsylvania 18766-0003
800-945-5378
www.wilkes.edu/academics/colleges/science-and-engineering
/biology-health-sciences/health-sciences
/premedical-programs.aspx

NAME OF PROGRAM
Guthrie or WVHCS Premedical Scholars Program

LENGTH OF PROGRAM
8 years

APPLICATION DEADLINE
November 15

INFORMATION ABOUT THE PROGRAM
This program is specifically for students who come from rural or underserved areas of Pennsylvania. Students must be committed to a career in primary health medicine. Students may major in any subject.

TRANSFER STUDENTS CONSIDERED
No

CITIZENSHIP REQUIREMENTS
U.S. citizen or permanent resident visa; must be from a rural or medically underserved area of Pennsylvania

MINIMUM REQUIRED FACTORS IN SELECTION

CLASSES

No specific requirement

GPA

Top ten percent of high school class

SAT

1,250 critical reading and math

ACT

No specific requirement

ACCEPTANCES

Two students are accepted each year.

FACTORS REQUIRED TO CONTINUE IN PROGRAM

3.5 overall and science GPA

MCAT REQUIRED

Yes; minimum score equal to previous year's average of incoming class; for 2010 that score was a 30 with no sub-score below 9

FINANCIAL AID

No special financial aid for students in the program.

COST

	Resident Tuition and Fees ($)	Non Resident Tuition and Fees ($)
Undergraduate	32,356	not applicable
Medical school	46,952	not applicable

COLLEGE
Temple University

MEDICAL SCHOOL
Temple University School of Medicine

ADDRESS
Temple University
Office of Admission
1801 North Broad Street
Philadelphia, Pennsylvania 19122
215-204-7200
www.temple.edu/healthadvising/healthscholars.html
healthadvising@temple.edu

NAME OF PROGRAM
Pre-Med Health Scholar Program

LENGTH OF PROGRAM
7 or 8 years

APPLICATION DEADLINE
December 18 for the Pre-Med Health Scholar Program

INFORMATION ABOUT THE PROGRAM
Students are first required to apply to the undergraduate college
at Temple before submitting an application to the Pre-Med Health
Scholar Program. Students must be admitted to Temple and the
honors college before the Pre-Med Health Scholar deadline.

To be considered for the seven-year program, applicants admitted to the Pre-Med Health Scholar Program must submit an
additional application during their first semester at Temple. Decisions on the accelerated program will be made based on first
semester grades.

The application requires three letters of recommendation, a
high school transcript to both the undergraduate college and the
Pre-Med program, and a demonstrated commitment to service
and volunteer opportunities.

TRANSFER STUDENTS CONSIDERED
No

CITIZENSHIP REQUIREMENTS

U.S. citizen or permanent resident visa

MINIMUM REQUIRED FACTORS IN SELECTION

CLASSES

Four years of high school math and science

GPA

3.8; average GPA of accepted Health Scholars was 4.00.

SAT

1,350 critical reading and math. Average SAT of accepted Health Scholars was 740 critical reading, 750 math.

ACT

32. Average ACT of accepted Health Scholars was 32.

ACCEPTANCES

In 2015, the program recieved 127 applications, interviewed 36 applicants, and accepted 15 students.

FACTORS REQUIRED TO CONTINUE IN PROGRAM

3.5 overall and science GPA with no more than one undergraduate grade of C and no failed courses

MCAT REQUIRED

Yes; minimum 70th percentile in each section on the new MCAT

FINANCIAL AID

No special financial aid for students in the program

COST

	Resident Tuition and Fees ($)	Non Resident Tuition and Fees ($)
Undergraduate	15,188	25,494
Medical school	48,452	54,258

COLLEGE

Washington & Jefferson College

MEDICAL SCHOOL

Temple University School of Medicine

ADDRESS

Washington & Jefferson College
Office of Admission
60 South Lincoln Street
Washington, Pennsylvania 15301-4812
724-223-6025
https://www.washjeff.edu
/pre-health-professions-school-affiliations
prehealth@washjeff.edu

NAME OF PROGRAM

Medical Scholars Program

LENGTH OF PROGRAM

8 years

APPLICATION DEADLINE

As early in the fall as possible for Washington & Jefferson; January 1 for the Medical Scholars Program

INFORMATION ABOUT THE PROGRAM

Students first apply to Washington & Jefferson and after being accepted apply to the Medical Scholars Program. Washington & Jefferson interviews students before deciding which students to recommend to Temple. Temple also interviews students in whom they have an interest. Students are required to complete over 50 hours of healthcare experience and show a demonstrated commitment to community service. Students may apply to other medical schools but will lose their guaranteed seat if they do so.

TRANSFER STUDENTS CONSIDERED

No

CITIZENSHIP REQUIREMENTS

U.S. citizen or permanent resident visa.

MINIMUM REQUIRED FACTORS IN SELECTION

CLASSES

No specific requirement although AP science coursework is expected.

GPA

Top five percent of the student's high school class

SAT

1,350 critical reading and math; no section under 600, including writing

ACT

31

ACCEPTANCES

No information provided

FACTORS REQUIRED TO CONTINUE IN PROGRAM

3.5 overall and science GPA with no grade less than a C

MCAT REQUIRED

Yes; minimum 70th percentile in each section on the new MCAT

FINANCIAL AID

No special financial aid for students in the program

COST

	Resident Tuition and Fees ($)	Non Resident Tuition and Fees ($)
Undergraduate	42,656	42,656
Medical school	48,452	54,258

COLLEGE

University of Pittsburgh

MEDICAL SCHOOL

University of Pittsburgh School of Medicine

ADDRESS

University of Pittsburgh
Office of Admissions and Financial Aid
4227 Fifth Avenue
Alumni Hall
Pittsburgh, Pennsylvania 15260-6601
412-624-7488
www.medadmissions.pitt.edu/admissions-requirements
/guaranteed-admissions.php
admissions@medschool.pitt.edu

NAME OF PROGRAM

Guaranteed admission

LENGTH OF PROGRAM

8 years

APPLICATION DEADLINE

December 1

INFORMATION ABOUT THE PROGRAM

Students interested in the program must indicate interest in pre-medicine or bioengineering on their undergraduate application. Students are required during the undergraduate years to continue medically related activities, including research and volunteer activities.

TRANSFER STUDENTS CONSIDERED

No

CITIZENSHIP REQUIREMENTS

U.S. citizen or permanent resident visa

MINIMUM REQUIRED FACTORS IN SELECTION

CLASSES

No specific requirement

GPA

Highest grade point average available

SAT

1,450 critical reading and math

ACT

33

ACCEPTANCES

In recent years they have accepted approximately 15 students.

FACTORS REQUIRED TO CONTINUE IN PROGRAM

3.75 overall and science GPA; must also engage in undergraduate research

MCAT REQUIRED

No, unless student wishes to be considered for merit scholarships or is applying to the MD/PhD program

FINANCIAL AID

No special financial aid for students in the program

COST

	Resident Tuition and Fees ($)	Non Resident Tuition and Fees ($)
Undergraduate	17,292	28,058
Medical school	50,852	52,306

COLLEGE

Inter American University of Puerto Rico at Ponce (UIA)

MEDICAL SCHOOL

Ponce School of Medicine

ADDRESS

Inter American University of Puerto Rico at Ponce
104 Turpo Industrial Park Road #1
Mercedita, PR 00715-1602
787-284-1912
www.psm.edu/Student_Affairs/Admissions/MD
/md_program_description.htm

NAME OF PROGRAM

Binary Programs

LENGTH OF PROGRAM

7 years

APPLICATION DEADLINE

December 15

INFORMATION ABOUT THE PROGRAM

The focus of the program is to educate physicians to provide medical care for Puerto Rico. In a recent class entering the medical school, seventy-seven percent of the students came from Puerto Rico and twenty-three percent from the continental U.S. Classes are held in both English and Spanish, so students need to be proficient in Spanish.

TRANSFER STUDENTS CONSIDERED

No

CITIZENSHIP REQUIREMENTS

U.S. citizen or permanent resident visa; residents of Puerto Rico are given preference

MINIMUM REQUIRED FACTORS IN SELECTION

None listed

ACCEPTANCES

No information provided

FACTORS REQUIRED TO CONTINUE IN PROGRAM

Overall GPA of 3.2 and a 3.0 science GPA; must maintain minimum 3.0 GPA each semester

MCAT REQUIRED

Yes; minimum score of 20

FINANCIAL AID

No special financial aid for students in the program

COST

	Resident Tuition and Fees ($)	Non Resident Tuition and Fees ($)
Undergraduate	4,852	4,852
Medical school	35,336	49,281

COLLEGE

Pontifical Catholic University of Puerto Rico (PUCPR)

MEDICAL SCHOOL

Ponce School of Medicine

ADDRESS

Pontifical Catholic University of Puerto Rico
2250 Las Americas Avenue, Suite 284
Ponce, PR 00717-9777
787-841-2000
www.psm.edu/Student_Affairs/Admissions/MD
/md_program_description.htm

NAME OF PROGRAM

Binary Programs

LENGTH OF PROGRAM

6 years

APPLICATION DEADLINE

December 15

INFORMATION ABOUT THE PROGRAM

The focus of the program is to educate physicians to provide medical care for Puerto Rico. In a recent class entering the medical school, seventy-seven percent of the students came from Puerto Rico and twenty-three percent from the continental U.S. Classes are held in both English and Spanish, so students need to be proficient in Spanish.

TRANSFER STUDENTS CONSIDERED

No

CITIZENSHIP REQUIREMENTS

U.S. citizen or permanent resident visa; residents of Puerto Rico are given preference

MINIMUM REQUIRED FACTORS IN SELECTION

None listed

ACCEPTANCES

No information provided

FACTORS REQUIRED TO CONTINUE IN PROGRAM

Overall GPA of 3.2 and a 3.0 science GPA; must maintain minimum 3.0 GPA each semester

MCAT REQUIRED

Yes; minimum score of 20

FINANCIAL AID

No special financial aid for students in the program

COST

	Resident Tuition and Fees ($)	Non Resident Tuition and Fees ($)
Undergraduate	5,000	5,000
Medical school	35,336	49,281

COLLEGE
Brown University

MEDICAL SCHOOL
Warren Alpert Medical School of Brown University

ADDRESS
PLME Office
Brown University
Box G-A222
91 Waterman Street
Providence, Rhode Island 02912-0001
401-863-9790
www.brown.edu/academics/medical/plme/
PLME@brown.edu

NAME OF PROGRAM
Program in Liberal Medical Education (PLME)

LENGTH OF PROGRAM
8 years

APPLICATION DEADLINE
January 1

INFORMATION ABOUT THE PROGRAM
Brown University has no distribution requirements, and this carries over to the PLME. Students may study any of the almost one hundred majors available at Brown. PLME encourages students to pursue their interests in depth, whether in the natural sciences, the humanities, or the social sciences. Students may extend their undergraduate program by a year or two to pursue additional academic interests. Students may also work on an additional graduate degree such as a PhD or MPH while pursuing the BS/MD.

In addition to academics, PLME is looking for students who have motivation, maturity, character, and intellectual breadth.

PLME has enrichment activities including opportunities to observe physicians working, the chance to have an international experience while at Brown, and research opportunities.

The early decision option at PLME is no longer available. PLME is unusual in that interviews at the medical school are not required. Brown University does encourage students to have an interview with an alumni interviewer for the college. If students are admitted to Brown undergraduate, their application is considered by the PLME committee.

Students can apply to other medical schools, but in doing so they will lose their guaranteed spot at the medical school.

TRANSFER STUDENTS CONSIDERED

No

CITIZENSHIP REQUIREMENTS

International students considered

MINIMUM REQUIRED FACTORS IN SELECTION

CLASSES

Recommended are four years of English, three years of math, three years of foreign language, two years of science above freshman level, two years of history, and one year of coursework in elective academic subjects.

GPA

No minimum; eighty-eight percent of admitted students in top five percent of high school class and most are in the top 1 percent.

SAT

No minimum; average SAT scores over the last five years were critical reading, 731; math, 741; and writing 746; two subject tests required, one of which should be a science subject test

ACT

May be substituted for SAT and SAT subject tests; writing section required

ACCEPTANCES

There were 2,290 applicants for the class of 2015; 90 students were offered admission; 61 matriculated into the program.

FACTORS REQUIRED TO CONTINUE IN PROGRAM

None listed

MCAT REQUIRED

No

FINANCIAL AID

Brown University meets one hundred percent of a student's financial need. Grants and loans are also available for the medical school.

COST

	Resident Tuition and Fees ($)	Non Resident Tuition and Fees ($)
Undergraduate	49,346	49,346
Medical school	53,416	53,416

COLLEGE
Grambling State University

MEDICAL SCHOOL
Meharry Medical College

ADDRESS
BS/MD Program Site Coordinator
Grambling State University
403 Main Street
Grambling, Louisiana 71245-2715
318-247-3811
www.gram.edu/academics/majors/arts-and-sciences
/biology/training.php
admissions@gram.edu

NAME OF PROGRAM
Bachelor of Science/Doctor of Medicine Program

LENGTH OF PROGRAM
7 or 8 years

APPLICATION DEADLINE
Not provided

INFORMATION ABOUT THE PROGRAM
This program is designed to increase the number of African
American physicians. Grambling and Meharry are both historically black colleges. Students may take seven or eight years to
complete the program. Students must also agree to participate
in a six-week summer program at the medical college designed to
enrich the academic and clinic experiences.

TRANSFER STUDENTS CONSIDERED
No

CITIZENSHIP REQUIREMENTS
U.S. citizen or permanent resident visa

MINIMUM REQUIRED FACTORS IN SELECTION

CLASSES
No specific requirement

GPA
3.25 overall and science GPA

SAT
900 critical reading and math

ACT
20

ACCEPTANCES
No information provided

FACTORS REQUIRED TO CONTINUE IN PROGRAM
None listed

MCAT REQUIRED
Not listed

FINANCIAL AID
Merit scholarships are available that may include full tuition.

COST

	Resident Tuition and Fees ($)	Non Resident Tuition and Fees ($)
Undergraduate	7,063	16,086
Medical school	50,098	50,098

COLLEGE
Baylor University

MEDICAL SCHOOL
Baylor College of Medicine

ADDRESS
Prehealth Studies Office
Baylor University
B.111 Baylor Science Building
One Bear Place #97341
Waco, Texas 76798-7341
254-710-3659
www.baylor.edu/prehealth/index.php?id=36430
B2B@baylor.edu

NAME OF PROGRAM
Guaranteed Admission Program/Baylor2 Medical Track

LENGTH OF PROGRAM
8 years

APPLICATION DEADLINE
November 1

INFORMATION ABOUT THE PROGRAM
Four years of college at Baylor University are required as part of
the program. Students are encouraged to study abroad or work
on a research project if they have time during their four years at
Baylor University. According to Baylor University, the program
is designed to offer the best students the "opportunity to broaden
their educational horizons." Students should list pre-medicine as
their pre-professional area of study on the Baylor application. Students who meet the basic admissions criteria will be invited to apply to the program. There are two interviews with this program.
The first, at Baylor University, will determine which students are
recommended for the Baylor College of Medicine. The College of
Medicine will conduct separate interviews with those students.

Baylor University and Baylor College of Medicine are not affiliated institutions. Baylor College of Medicine is a private non-
sectarian institution.

TRANSFER STUDENTS CONSIDERED
No

CITIZENSHIP REQUIREMENTS
U.S. citizen or permanent resident visa

MINIMUM REQUIRED FACTORS IN SELECTION

CLASSES

No specific requirement

GPA

3.7 unweighted or top five percent of high school class

SAT

1,400 critical reading and math

ACT

32

2009–2010 ACCEPTANCES

Six students are selected each year.

FACTORS REQUIRED TO CONTINUE IN PROGRAM

3.5 overall and science GPA. Student receiving top scholarship has required GPA of 3.7. No grades lower than C. Must complete a modified application to Baylor College of Medicine.

MCAT REQUIRED

Yes; scores should fall in the 500–507 range with no section score less than 125.

FINANCIAL AID

Grants, loans, and work study available for undergraduates. Limited financial aid for medical school. One student will receive a scholarship of $10,000 per year for all eight years.

COST

	Resident Tuition and Fees ($)	Non Resident Tuition and Fees ($)
Undergraduate	40,738	40,738
Medical school	18,536	31,618

COLLEGE

Rice University

MEDICAL SCHOOL

Baylor College of Medicine

ADDRESS

Rice University
Admission Office-MS 17
6100 South Main Street
Houston, Texas 77005-1827
713-348-7423
http://futureowls.rice.edu/medical_scholars_program.asp
admission@rice.edu

NAME OF PROGRAM

Medical Scholars Program

LENGTH OF PROGRAM

8 years

APPLICATION DEADLINE

December 1

INFORMATION ABOUT THE PROGRAM

"The Medical Scholars Program promotes the education of students who are scientifically competent, compassionate, and socially conscious." This is the stated goal of the program between Rice University and Baylor College of Medicine.

Students in this program are encouraged to explore all of the options available to Rice undergraduates. Explorations of the liberal arts and the student's own interests are also encouraged.

Students may apply to Rice regular decision or early decision. Those applying early decision must do so by the early decision date of November 1. If a student applies early decision and is admitted, they must commit to Rice by January 1 even though decisions by the Baylor College of Medicine will not be announced until late April. Rice will notify finalists in March, and Baylor conducts interviews in April. Students applying to the Rice/Baylor program may not apply to any of the other Baylor medical scholars programs.

The program is not binding, and students may apply out to other medical schools.

TRANSFER STUDENTS CONSIDERED

No

CITIZENSHIP REQUIREMENTS
International students considered

MINIMUM REQUIRED FACTORS IN SELECTION

CLASSES
No specific requirement

GPA
No specific requirement; typical students in top five percent of high school class

SAT
No specific requirement; mid-range scores of students entering Rice, 1,350–1,510. Students must take two SAT subject tests, which should relate to your area of study.

ACT
No specific requirement, although SAT subject tests are not required if a student takes the ACT.

ACCEPTANCES
Six students are selected each year. For the 2015 class, 2,544 applicants applied, 287 were admitted to Rice, 37 students interviewed with Baylor College of Medicine.

FACTORS REQUIRED TO CONTINUE IN PROGRAM
None listed

MCAT REQUIRED
Yes. Required score under new MCAT has not yet been determined.

FINANCIAL AID
Rice covers one hundred percent of a student's financial need. This makes available substantial financial aid to families with lower income levels. Like most medical schools, financial aid at Baylor is limited.

COST

	Resident Tuition and Fees ($)	Non Resident Tuition and Fees ($)
Undergraduate	42,253	42,253
Medical school	18,536	31,618

COLLEGE
University of Houston

MEDICAL SCHOOL
Baylor College of Medicine

ADDRESS
Dean of Instruction
DeBakey High School for Health Professions
3100 Shenandoah
Houston, TX 77021
713-741-2410
www.houstonisd.org/domain/3328

NAME OF PROGRAM
Houston Premedical Academy

LENGTH OF PROGRAM
8 years

APPLICATION DEADLINE
Early February. The date changes each year, so please check carefully.

INFORMATION ABOUT THE PROGRAM
This program is open to students of the Michael E. DeBakey High School for Health Professions only. Three applications are required, including one to the University of Houston, one to the University of Houston Honors College, and one to the Houston Premedical Academy. Students are admitted to the Honors College at the University of Houston and may major in any subject. A Medicine and Society minor is expected regardless of the major. Students in the program spend their summers in activities related to health care issues.

TRANSFER STUDENTS CONSIDERED
No

CITIZENSHIP REQUIREMENTS
U.S. citizen or permanent resident visa

MINIMUM REQUIRED FACTORS IN SELECTION

CLASSES
No specific requirement

GPA
3.5 overall, and a core GPA of at least 3.2, including math, science, and English

SAT
580 critical reading, 600 math, and 520 writing

ACT
Not considered

ACCEPTANCES
Up to 6 students are selected each year.

FACTORS REQUIRED TO CONTINUE IN PROGRAM
3.5 overall and science GPA; no grade lower than a C in required classes

MCAT REQUIRED
Yes; minimum score of 500–507 on the new MCAT, with no section score less than 125

FINANCIAL AID
All students in the program will receive scholarship support.

COST

	Resident Tuition and Fees ($)	Non Resident Tuition and Fees ($)
Undergraduate	10,704	not applicable
Medical school	18,536	not applicable

COLLEGE

University of Texas Pan American

MEDICAL SCHOOL

Baylor College of Medicine

ADDRESS

UTPA, Biology Department
1201 West University Drive
Edinburg, Texas 78539-2909
956-316-7025
http://portal.utpa.edu/utpa_main/daa_home/cose_home
/biology_home/biology_jp/jp_pmh
cindy@utpa.edu

NAME OF PROGRAM

Premedical Honors College

LENGTH OF PROGRAM

8 years

APPLICATION DEADLINE

Deadline varies but generally near the end of January or early
February

INFORMATION ABOUT THE PROGRAM

The University of Texas at Brownsville and the University of
Texas Pan American are being merged into one new university,
the University of Texas Rio Grande Valley. It is not know at this
time what effect this will have on these BS/MD programs.

The goal of this program is to increase the number of physicians serving the medically underserved area of South Texas. Students are required to major in biology, chemistry, or biochemistry
and minor in one of the other sciences. Students complete two applications including one to the undergraduate college and one to
the premedical honors college.

TRANSFER STUDENTS CONSIDERED

No

CITIZENSHIP REQUIREMENTS

U.S. citizen or permanent resident visa; residence in South Texas

MINIMUM REQUIRED FACTORS IN SELECTION

CLASSES

No specific requirement

GPA

No specific requirement

SAT

No minimum score, but applicants must take the SAT

ACT

Not accepted.

ACCEPTANCES

No information provided

FACTORS REQUIRED TO CONTINUE IN PROGRAM

3.2 science GPA and 3.4 overall GPA, with no grade lower than a C

MCAT REQUIRED

Yes; minimum score 28 with no sub-score below 8

FINANCIAL AID

No special financial aid for students in the program

COST

	Resident Tuition and Fees ($)	Non Resident Tuition and Fees ($)
Undergraduate	6,134	not applicable
Medical school	28,536	not applicable

COLLEGE

Prairie View A & M University; South Texas College; Tarleton State University; Texas A & M International University; Texas A & M University at College Station; Texas A & M University at Commerce; Texas A & M University at Corpus Christi; Texas A & M University at Kingsville; West Texas A & M University

MEDICAL SCHOOL

Texas A & M Health Science Center College of Medicine

ADDRESS

Texas A&M Health Science Center College of Medicine
Office of Admissions
Partnership for Primary Care
8447 State Highway 47
Bryan, Texas 77807-3260
979-436-0233
http://medicine.tamhsc.edu/admissions/ppc/
COM-PPC@medicine.tamhsc.edu

NAME OF PROGRAM

Partnership for Primary Care

LENGTH OF PROGRAM

8 years

APPLICATION DEADLINE

February 1

INFORMATION ABOUT THE PROGRAM

This program is designed to help train students from rural areas of Texas that are facing a physician shortage. The focus of the program is training students in primary care medicine who will return to their home areas to practice medicine. Various medical enrichment activities are made available to students in the program, including workshops on success in medical school, medical seminars, and meetings with other students in the program. There are also summer enrichment programs that students participate in as well as opportunities for doctor shadowing.

TRANSFER STUDENTS CONSIDERED

No

CITIZENSHIP REQUIREMENTS

U.S. citizen or permanent resident visa; resident of Texas; legal residence in a rural or underserved area or health professions shortage area as defined by the Health Professions Resource Center, Texas Department of Health

MINIMUM REQUIRED FACTORS IN SELECTION

CLASSES

No specific requirement

GPA

3.5 unweighted, and a preference for students in the top 10 percent of high school class

SAT

1,200 on critical reading and math

ACT

26

2009–2010 ACCEPTANCES

No information provided

FACTORS REQUIRED TO CONTINUE IN PROGRAM

3.25 GPA after freshman year and a 3.5 cumulative GPA in subsequent years; can have no grade in required courses below a C

MCAT REQUIRED

Yes; minimum score of 500 on the new MCAT, with no section score less than 125

FINANCIAL AID

No special financial aid for students in the program

COST

	Resident Tuition and Fees ($)	Non Resident Tuition and Fees ($)
Undergraduate	9,745	not applicable
Medical school	16,432	not applicable

COLLEGE

Texas Tech University

MEDICAL SCHOOL

Texas Tech University Health Sciences Center
School of Medicine

ADDRESS

Texas Tech University Health Sciences Center
School of Medicine Office of Admissions 2B116
3601 4th Street MS 6216
Lubbock, Texas 79430-6216
806-743-2297
www.ttuhsc.edu/som/admissions/umsi.aspx
Linda.Prado@ttuhsc.edu

NAME OF PROGRAM

Undergraduate to Medical School Initiative

LENGTH OF PROGRAM

8 years

APPLICATION DEADLINE

December 1 for the application to the program

INFORMATION ABOUT THE PROGRAM

Students apply to the undergraduate college and the honors college and must be admitted before applying to the program. It takes four to six weeks for the undergraduate application to be processed, so students should plan on getting their undergraduate application submitted in early October. Must be a high school senior when applying to the program. Any study abroad program taken must be affiliated with Texas Tech University.

TRANSFER STUDENTS CONSIDERED

No

CITIZENSHIP REQUIREMENTS

U.S. citizen or permanent resident visa; Texas resident

MINIMUM REQUIRED FACTORS IN SELECTION

CLASSES
No specific requirements

GPA
3.70 unweighted; preference given to students ranking in the top
ten percent of their class

SAT
1,300 critical reading and math

ACT
29

ACCEPTANCES
No information provided

FACTORS REQUIRED TO CONTINUE IN PROGRAM
Science GPA of 3.6 and overall GPA of 3.7. A grade of B must be
earned in all prerequisite courses.

MCAT REQUIRED
No

FINANCIAL AID
No special financial aid for students in the program

COST

	Resident Tuition and Fees ($)	Non Resident Tuition and Fees ($)
Undergraduate	7,984	not applicable
Medical school	14,471	not applicable

COLLEGE

The University of Texas at San Antonio

MEDICAL SCHOOL

The University of Texas Health Science Center at San Antonio

ADDRESS

The University of Texas at San Antonio
One UTSA Circle
San Antonio, Texas 78249-1644
210-458-4011
www.utsystem.edu/initiatives/time/fame.html

NAME OF PROGRAM

Facilitated Access to Medical Education (FAME)

LENGTH OF PROGRAM

7 years

APPLICATION DEADLINE

December 1, although the program recommends November 1.
Must be admitted to UTSA by December 1.

INFORMATION ABOUT THE PROGRAM

In response to the University of Texas System Request for Proposals to develop innovative and fully integrated pilot programs which lead to the award of both baccalaureate and Doctor of Medicine degrees, the University of Texas Health Science Center at San Antonio (UTHSCSA) and the University of Texas at San Antonio (UTSA) have partnered to implement an innovative program.

In order to meet degree requirements set for all college graduates in the State of Texas, core courses have been interwoven into a fully functional, collaborative seven- year curriculum with the end result of graduating physicians (Facilitated Acceptance to Medical Education [FAME] Program). This shared project uses traditional course structure, team-taught courses, and innovative seminar courses structured around disease-related experiences. The program was carefully developed to provide opportunities for students to exit the program should their interests take them to any number of other health-related fields.

Students must complete two applications including a University of Texas application and a FAME application.

TRANSFER STUDENTS CONSIDERED

No

CITIZENSHIP REQUIREMENTS

U.S. citizen or permanent resident visa; resident of Texas

MINIMUM REQUIRED FACTORS IN SELECTION

CLASSES

No specific requirement

GPA

3.6 science and overall GPA on a 4.0 scale or a 91 science and overall GPA on a 100 point scale

SAT

1,300 critical reading and math with minimum of 650 on each section

ACT

29 with a minimum of 29 on both the English and Math sections

ACCEPTANCES

No information provided

FACTORS REQUIRED TO CONTINUE IN PROGRAM

3.4 overall and science GPA

MCAT REQUIRED

Yes; 27 with no subscore less than 8 on the old MCAT

FINANCIAL AID

No special financial aid for students in the program

COST

	Resident Tuition and Fees ($)	Non Resident Tuition and Fees ($)
Undergraduate	9,361	not applicable
Medical school	20,964	not applicable

COLLEGE

The University of Texas at Dallas

MEDICAL SCHOOL

The University of Texas Southwestern Medical Center at Dallas

ADDRESS

Health Professions Advising Office
The University of Texas at Dallas
800 West Campbell Road
Richardson, Texas 75080-3021
972-883-2111
www.utdallas.edu/pre-health/ut-pact
ut-pact@utdallas.edu

NAME OF PROGRAM

UT-PACT BS/MD Program

LENGTH OF PROGRAM

7 years

APPLICATION DEADLINE

December 1

INFORMATION ABOUT THE PROGRAM

This is a pilot program as part of the initiative of the University of Texas to provide streamlined and better access to medical education to residents of Texas. Applicants are required to have a letter of recommendation from a high school guidance counselor and a high school math or science teacher and an additional letter of character reference, ideally from a health care professional. Students must be admitted to the undergraduate college before applying to the program; it takes about one month for applications to be processed. Early applications are encouraged. Students will be notified of their status in the program by April 15.

TRANSFER STUDENTS CONSIDERED

No

CITIZENSHIP REQUIREMENTS

U.S. citizen or permanent resident visa; resident of Texas

MINIMUM REQUIRED FACTORS IN SELECTION

CLASSES

No specific requirement

GPA

3.5 unweighted GPA, average GPA of students attending the program is 3.96

SAT

Minimum 550 critical reading and 550 math; average SAT score of students attending the program is 1,519 critical reading and math.

ACT

27; average ACT of students attending the program is 35.

ACCEPTANCES

No information provided

FACTORS REQUIRED TO CONTINUE IN PROGRAM

Overall and science GPA of 3.5

MCAT REQUIRED

No

FINANCIAL AID

No special financial aid for students in the program

COST

	Resident Tuition and Fees ($)	Non Resident Tuition and Fees ($)
Undergraduate	11,806	not applicable
Medical school	7,913	not applicable

COLLEGE

St. Mary's University; Texas A & M International University; University of Texas (UT) Pan American

MEDICAL SCHOOL

University of Texas Health Science Center at San Antonio

ADDRESS

Director of Admissions and Special Programs
School of Medicine
The University of Texas Health Science Center at San Antonio
7703 Floyd Curl Drive
San Antonio, Texas 78229-3900
210-567-6080
http://som.uthscsa.edu/Admissions
/earlyMatriculationProgram.asp
chapab@uthscsa.edu

NAME OF PROGRAM

Facilitated Admissions for South Texas Scholars (FASTS)

LENGTH OF PROGRAM

7 or 8 years

APPLICATION DEADLINE

February 1

INFORMATION ABOUT THE PROGRAM

Students receive mentoring from medical school faculty as well as enrichment and clinical experiences in a Summer Premedical Academy. Students are expected to complete a biology or chemistry degree at one of the colleges. There is also an MCAT review course during the summer after junior year in college.

TRANSFER STUDENTS CONSIDERED

Yes

CITIZENSHIP REQUIREMENTS

U.S. citizen or permanent resident visa; Texas resident

MINIMUM REQUIRED FACTORS IN SELECTION

None listed

ACCEPTANCES

No information provided

FACTORS REQUIRED TO CONTINUE IN PROGRAM

Overall and science GPA of 3.25 with no grade lower than a C

MCAT REQUIRED

Yes; ratio of GPA/MCAT will determine if student advances: students with ratio of 3.5/29–3.75/27, with no subsection score below a 7 are eligible for acceptance to the medical school. A minimum score in the 75th percentile is anticipated with the new MCAT.

FINANCIAL AID

No special financial aid for students in the program

COST

	Resident Tuition and Fees ($)	Non Resident Tuition and Fees ($)
Undergraduate	varies by college	not applicable
Medical school	20,964	not applicable

COLLEGE

Prairie View A & M University; Texas A & M International University; Texas Southern University; The University of Texas Rio Grande Valley; The University of Texas at El Paso

MEDICAL SCHOOL

University of Texas Medical Branch at Galveston

ADDRESS

Director, Medical School Enrichment Programs
University of Texas Medical Branch
301 University Boulevard
Galveston, Texas 77555-0807
409-772-1212
www.utmb.edu/somenrichprograms/
ldcain@utmb.edu

NAME OF PROGRAM

Early Medical School Acceptance Program (EMSAP)

LENGTH OF PROGRAM

8 years

APPLICATION DEADLINE

January 31

INFORMATION ABOUT THE PROGRAM

Students participate in a summer enrichment program on the medical school campus that provides clinical exposure to the medical field. Students major in biology or chemistry. They will have continued clinical exposure during their four years of undergraduate study. An MCAT prep course is part of the program. These programs are aimed specifically to increase the number of Latino and Latina physicians.

TRANSFER STUDENTS CONSIDERED

No

CITIZENSHIP REQUIREMENTS

U.S. citizen or permanent resident visa; Texas residents only

MINIMUM REQUIRED FACTORS IN SELECTION

CLASSES

No specific requirement

GPA

3.25

SAT

1,500 on critical reading, math, and writing

ACT

21

ACCEPTANCES

No information provided

FACTORS REQUIRED TO CONTINUE IN PROGRAM

3.25 GPA

MCAT REQUIRED

Yes; minimum score 498

FINANCIAL AID

No special financial aid for students in program

COST

	Resident Tuition and Fees ($)	Non Resident Tuition and Fees ($)
Undergraduate	varies by college	not applicable
Medical school	17,589	not applicable

COLLEGE

The University of Texas Rio Grande Valley; The University of Texas at El Paso; The University of Texas-Pan American at Edinburg

MEDICAL SCHOOL

University of Texas Medical Branch at Galveston; University of Texas Medical School–Houston

ADDRESS

Director, A-PRIME TIME
University of Texas Rio Grande Valley
One West University Boulevard
Brownsville, Texas 78520
888-882-4026
http://aprimetime.org/
aprimetime@utrgv.edu

The University of Texas at El Paso
500 West University Avenue
Office for Undergraduate Studies
Mike Loya Academic Services Bldg. Rm. 218
El Paso, TX 79968
http://aprimetime.org/
aprimetime@utrgv.edu

NAME OF PROGRAM

A-PRIME TIME

LENGTH OF PROGRAM

6 years

APPLICATION DEADLINE

January 31

INFORMATION ABOUT THE PROGRAM

This program is unique because it includes three years of undergraduate study and three years of medical school. Students apply to only one of the undergraduate colleges and indicate an interest in the Pre-Health Professions Program. Students participate in a summer enrichment program on the medical school campus that provides clinical exposure to the medical field. An MCAT prep course is part of the program.

TRANSFER STUDENTS CONSIDERED

No

CITIZENSHIP REQUIREMENTS

U.S. citizen or permanent resident visa; Texas resident

MINIMUM REQUIRED FACTORS IN SELECTION

CLASSES

No specific requirement

GPA

3.25 science and cumulative

SAT

1,500 on critical reading, math, and writing

ACT

21

ACCEPTANCES

No information provided

FFACTORS REQUIRED TO CONTINUE IN PROGRAM

3.5 overall and science GPA

MCAT REQUIRED

Yes; minimum score not provided

FINANCIAL AID

No special financial aid for students in program

COST

	Resident Tuition and Fees ($)	Non Resident Tuition and Fees ($)
Undergraduate	varies by college	not applicable
Medical school	7,589	not applicable

COLLEGE
Virginia Commonwealth University

MEDICAL SCHOOL
Virginia Commonwealth University School of Medicine

ADDRESS
Virginia Commonwealth University
The Honors College
701 West Grace Street
Richmond, Virginia 23284-3010
804-828-1803
https://www.pubapps.vcu.edu/honors/guaranteed/medicine
/index.aspx
honors@vcu.edu

NAME OF PROGRAM
Guaranteed Admission Program (Medicine)

LENGTH OF PROGRAM
8 years

APPLICATION DEADLINE
November 15

INFORMATION ABOUT THE PROGRAM
Two applications are required for this program, an application for
undergraduate admissions and an application for The Honors College Guaranteed Admission Program (Medicine). Students most
commonly major in biology or biomedical engineering, although
other majors are possible. There are a number of required science
courses for this program, so other majors require careful planning. Students must complete 120 hours of patient care related experience each year during the first three years of the program and
sixty additional hours the fourth year. Students are also expected
to complete ten hours of non-healthcare community service each
semester. During the third year of the program, students complete
a one-semester mentorship with a faculty member of the medical
school. Accepted students have an average of 450 hours of health
care related experience.

TRANSFER STUDENTS CONSIDERED
No

CITIZENSHIP REQUIREMENTS
U.S. citizen or permanent resident visa; Canadian residents also
considered; preference is given to Virginia residents.

MINIMUM REQUIRED FACTORS IN SELECTION

CLASSES

Four years of English, three years of math, three years of science, and three years of history or social studies; three years of a foreign language are strongly encouraged.

GPA

3.5 unweighted; average GPA of accepted students, 3.88 unweighted

SAT

1,270 on critical reading and math, with no sub-score below 530; average SAT score of accepted students, 1,490 with a range of 1,300 to 1,600

ACT

29; note that SAT is preferred but the ACT will be accepted.

ACCEPTANCES

In 2015, 34 students were accepted from a pool of approximately 400.

FACTORS REQUIRED TO CONTINUE IN PROGRAM

Cumulative and science GPA of 3.5; graduate with university honors

MCAT REQUIRED

Yes. Minimum score of 502

FINANCIAL AID

No special financial aid for students in the program

COST

	Resident Tuition and Fees ($)	Non Resident Tuition and Fees ($)
Undergraduate	10,951	26,535
Medical school	32,113	49,818

COLLEGE

Marshall University

MEDICAL SCHOOL

Marshall University Joan C. Edwards School of Medicine

ADDRESS

Marshall University
One John Marshall Drive
Huntington, West Virginia 25755
800-642-3463
http://jcesom.marshall.edu/students/accelerated-bsmd-program/
BSMDprogram@marshall.edu

NAME OF PROGRAM

Accelerated BS/MD Program

LENGTH OF PROGRAM

7 years

APPLICATION DEADLINE

January 8

INFORMATION ABOUT THE PROGRAM

Students in the program must major in biology and have the option of participating in honors programs. Students are also required to actively participate in various enrichment activities during the undergraduate years. Three letters of recommendation are required for admission to the program.

TRANSFER STUDENTS CONSIDERED

No

CITIZENSHIP REQUIREMENTS

U.S. citizen or permanent resident visa. West Virginia resident.

MINIMUM REQUIRED FACTORS IN SELECTION

CLASSES

No specific requirements

GPA

3.75 unweighted GPA

SAT

1,330 on critical reading and math and minimum math score of 610

ACT

30 composite with minimum math score of 27

ACCEPTANCES

No information provided

FACTORS REQUIRED TO CONTINUE IN PROGRAM

Overall GPA of 3.5

MCAT REQUIRED

No

FINANCIAL AID

Tuition waiver for the medical school portion

COST

	Resident Tuition and Fees ($)	Non Resident Tuition and Fees ($)
Undergraduate	6,814	Not applicable
Medical school	0	Not applicable

COLLEGE

Caldwell College

MEDICAL SCHOOL

American University of Antigua College of Medicine

ADDRESS

Caldwell College
Office of Health Professions Program
Department of NAtural and Physical Sciences
203 Raymond Hall
Caldwell University
120 Bloomfield Ave
Caldwell, New Jersey 07006-5310
973-618-3595
www.caldwell.edu/health-professions/affiliation-programs
Vukachukwu@caldwell.edu

NAME OF PROGRAM

Health Professions Affiliation Program Medicine

LENGTH OF PROGRAM

8 years

APPLICATION DEADLINE

January 15

INFORMATION ABOUT THE PROGRAM

Students can major in any topic.

TRANSFER STUDENTS CONSIDERED

No

CITIZENSHIP REQUIREMENTS

U.S. citizen or permanent resident visa

MINIMUM REQUIRED FACTORS IN SELECTION

CLASSES

No specific requirements

GPA

3.5 unweighted

SAT

1,200 critical reading and math

ACT

26

ACCEPTANCES

No information provided

FACTORS REQUIRED TO CONTINUE IN PROGRAM

No information provided

MCAT REQUIRED

No information provided.

FINANCIAL AID

No special financial aid for students in the program

COST

	Resident Tuition and Fees ($)	Non Resident Tuition and Fees ($)
Undergraduate	31,200	31,200
Medical school	35,000	35,000

COLLEGE
New Jersey Institute of Technology

MEDICAL SCHOOL
American University of Antigua College of Medicine

ADDRESS
Honors College
New Jersey Institute of Technology
University Heights
Newark, New Jersey 07102-1982
973-642-7664
http://honors.njit.edu/academics/acceleratedprograms
/PreHealthCareers.php
honors@njit.edu

NAME OF PROGRAM
Accelerated Medical Program

LENGTH OF PROGRAM
7 years

APPLICATION DEADLINE
November 15

INFORMATION ABOUT THE PROGRAM
Students must first be admitted to the honors college. Students spend their first three years at the New Jersey Institute of Technology, the next two years in Antigua, and the final two years at St. Michael's Medical Center adjoining NJIT.

Students may pursue any major. However biology; biomedical engineering; biochemistry; biophysics; mathematics; and science, technology, and society are preferred majors.

TRANSFER STUDENTS CONSIDERED
No

CITIZENSHIP REQUIREMENTS
U.S. citizen or permanent resident visa

MINIMUM REQUIRED FACTORS IN SELECTION

CLASSES
No specific requirements

GPA
Top 10 percent

SAT
1,400

ACT
32

ACCEPTANCES
No information provided

FACTORS REQUIRED TO CONTINUE IN PROGRAM
No information provided

MCAT REQUIRED
Yes. Test results do not affect admissions.

FINANCIAL AID
No special financial aid for students in the program

COST

	Resident Tuition and Fees ($)	Non Resident Tuition and Fees ($)
Undergraduate	16,108	30,326
Medical school	35,000	35,000

COLLEGE

Caldwell College

MEDICAL SCHOOL

St. George's University School of Medicine—
Grenada, West Indies

ADDRESS

Office of Health Professions Program
Department of NAtural and Physical Sciences
203 Raymond Hall
Caldwell University
120 Bloomfield Ave
Caldwell, New Jersey 07006-5310
973-618-3595
www.caldwell.edu/health-professions/affiliation-programs
Vukachukwu@caldwell.edu

NAME OF PROGRAM

Health Professions Affiliation Program Medicine

LENGTH OF PROGRAM

7 years

APPLICATION DEADLINE

January 15

INFORMATION ABOUT THE PROGRAM

Students spend their first three years at Caldwell and then complete four years at St. George's University, obtaining their BA after the first year of medical school. Students can major in any topic.

TRANSFER STUDENTS CONSIDERED

No

CITIZENSHIP REQUIREMENTS

U.S. citizen or permanent resident visa

MINIMUM REQUIRED FACTORS IN SELECTION

CLASSES

No specific requirements

GPA

3.5 unweighted

SAT

1,200 critical reading and math

ACT

26

ACCEPTANCES

No information provided

FACTORS REQUIRED TO CONTINUE IN PROGRAM

No information provided

MCAT REQUIRED

No information provided.

FINANCIAL AID

No special financial aid for students in the program

COST

	Resident Tuition and Fees ($)	Non Resident Tuition and Fees ($)
Undergraduate	31,200	31,200
Medical school	53,450	53,450

COLLEGE

New Jersey Institute of Technology

MEDICAL SCHOOL

St. George's University School of Medicine—
Grenada, West Indies

ADDRESS

Honors College
New Jersey Institute of Technology
University Heights
Newark, New Jersey 07102-1982
973-642-7664
http://honors.njit.edu/admission/pre-health-law/health.php
honors@njit.edu

NAME OF PROGRAM

Accelerated Medical Program

LENGTH OF PROGRAM

7 years

APPLICATION DEADLINE

November 15

INFORMATION ABOUT THE PROGRAM

Students must first be admitted to the honors college. Students
spend their first three years at the New Jersey Institute of Technology, the next two years in Grenada and the final two years at
St. Michael's Medical Center adjoining NJIT.

Applicants must provide evidence of their knowledge of a career in medicine through volunteering, shadowing, research, or
other related experiences.

Students may pursue any major. However biology; biomedical
engineering; biochemistry; biophysics; mathematics; and science,
technology, and society are preferred majors.

TRANSFER STUDENTS CONSIDERED

No

CITIZENSHIP REQUIREMENTS

International students considered

MINIMUM REQUIRED FACTORS IN SELECTION

CLASSES

No specific requirements

GPA

Top 10 percent

SAT

1,400 math and critical reading from a single sitting

ACT

30

ACCEPTANCES

No information provided

FACTORS REQUIRED TO CONTINUE IN PROGRAM

No information provided

MCAT REQUIRED

Yes; test results do not affect admissions.

FINANCIAL AID

No special financial aid for students in the program

COST

	Resident Tuition and Fees ($)	Non Resident Tuition and Fees ($)
Undergraduate	16,108	30,326
Medical school	53,450	53,450

BS/DO Programs by State

The information provided in the appendix is believed to be accurate as of the date of the publication of this book. However, BS/DO programs are constantly being started while others are being discontinued. Also, the information regarding minimal grades and test scores as well as the dates applications are required are subject to change at any time. If you find a program in which you have an interest, go to the website of that program to verify information. For updated information you can check our website: www.collegeadmissionspartners.com/bsmd-admissions/.

There is some inconsistency in the way GPA and test scores are reported. Some schools list only their minimum requirements. Some list the averages for *accepted* students. Others list the averages for *enrolled* students. These two averages are not interchangeable. Typically the averages for accepted students are higher than those for enrolled students.

COLLEGE

Pitzer College

MEDICAL SCHOOL

Western University of Health Sciences

ADDRESS

Pitzer College
Office of Admissions and Financial Aid
1050 N Mills Avenue
Claremont, California 91711
909-621-8129
http://pitweb.pitzer.edu/admission/joint-medical-program/
admission@pitzer.edu

NAME OF PROGRAM

Joint Medical Program

LENGTH OF PROGRAM

7 years

APPLICATION DEADLINE

January 1

INFORMATION ABOUT THE PROGRAM

Students interested in the program should have strong demonstrated community involvement, especially in health care fields,
and a desire to pursue primary care medicine. Students are encouraged to explore a wide variety of academic fields and may
major in any subject. During their time at Western University of
Health Sciences, students have the opportunity to gain experience
abroad by doing an international rotation.

TRANSFER STUDENTS CONSIDERED

No

CITIZENSHIP REQUIREMENTS

U.S. citizen or permanent resident visa

MINIMUM REQUIRED FACTORS IN SELECTION

CLASSES

Students should have taken advanced courses in biology, chemistry, physics, and calculus

GPA

No minimum requirement

SAT

No minimum requirement

ACT

No minimum requirement

ACCEPTANCES

A maximum of 6 students are accepted for this program per year.

FACTORS REQUIRED TO CONTINUE IN PROGRAM

None stated

MCAT REQUIRED

No

FINANCIAL AID

No special financial aid for students in the program

COST

	Resident Tuition and Fees ($)	Non Resident Tuition and Fees ($)
Undergraduate	48,670	48,670
Medical school	53,570	53,570

COLLEGE
Nova Southeastern University

MEDICAL SCHOOL
Nova Southeastern University

ADDRESS
Undergraduate Admissions
3301 College Avenue
Fort Lauderdale, Florida 33314-7796
954-262-8000
www.nova.edu/undergraduate/academics/dual-admission
/osteopathic-medicine.html
admissions@nova.edu

NAME OF PROGRAM
Dual Admission—Osteopathic Medicine

LENGTH OF PROGRAM
7 or 8 years

APPLICATION DEADLINE
January 1

INFORMATION ABOUT THE PROGRAM
Students may major in any subject that results in obtaining a BS.
Students applying to the program should have three letters of
recommendation including one from a science teacher, one from a
counselor, and one from a DO or an MD. Finalists will be invited
to interview at both the undergraduate and medical school at various dates between late January and early March.

TRANSFER STUDENTS CONSIDERED
No

CITIZENSHIP REQUIREMENTS
U.S. citizen or permanent resident visa

MINIMUM REQUIRED FACTORS IN SELECTION

CLASSES

Students should have taken four years of English and math (through pre-calculus), and four years of science including chemistry and biology (only three years of science required for eight-year program).

GPA

3.5

SAT

1,300 math and critical reading for seven-year program; 1,150 math and critical reading for eight-year program

ACT

29 for seven-year program; 25 for eight-year program

ACCEPTANCES

No information provided

FACTORS REQUIRED TO CONTINUE IN PROGRAM

Students must maintain an overall and science GPA of 3.3 for the seven-year program and 3.2 for the eight-year; no grade lower than a C+ in any prerequisite courses.

MCAT REQUIRED

Yes; 502 minimum with 125 minimum on all subsections

FINANCIAL AID

No special financial aid for students in the program

COST

	Resident Tuition and Fees ($)	Non Resident Tuition and Fees ($)
Undergraduate	26,910	26,910
Medical school	48,193	52,698

COLLEGE
Illinois Institute of Technology

MEDICAL SCHOOL
Midwestern University—Chicago College of Osteopathic
Medicine

ADDRESS
Office of Undergraduate Admission
10 W 33rd Street
Perlstein Hall, Room 101
Chicago, Illinois 60616
312-567-6941
http://admissions.iit.edu/undergraduate/programs
/dual-admission-osteopathic-medicine-bs-do
smeggs@iit.edu

NAME OF PROGRAM
Dual Admission Program

LENGTH OF PROGRAM
8 years

APPLICATION DEADLINE
December 15

INFORMATION ABOUT THE PROGRAM
The focus of this program is on preparing students in a technological field to prepare them for the increasing role of technology in medicine. The program requires an application to Illinois Institute of Technology and a supplemental application for the program as well as interviews with both IIT and the College of Medicine.

TRANSFER STUDENTS CONSIDERED
No

CITIZENSHIP REQUIREMENTS
U.S. citizen or permanent resident visa

MINIMUM REQUIRED FACTORS IN SELECTION

CLASSES

Students should have taken four years of English and math (through calculus), and three years of science including chemistry and physics

GPA

3.5, top 10% of class

SAT

1,400 math and critical reading

ACT

32

ACCEPTANCES

A maximum of 5–10 students are accepted for this program per year from approximately 20 finalists.

FACTORS REQUIRED TO CONTINUE IN PROGRAM

Students must maintain an overall GPA of 3.5.

MCAT REQUIRED

Yes; must score above the national average

FINANCIAL AID

No special financial aid for students in the program

COST

	Resident Tuition and Fees ($)	Non Resident Tuition and Fees ($)
Undergraduate	43,680	43,680
Medical school	50,131	55,567

COLLEGE

New York Institute of Technology; SUNY New Paltz; SUNY Old Westbury

MEDICAL SCHOOL

New York Institute of Technology College of Osteopathic Medicine

ADDRESS

New York Institute of Technology
Theobald Hall, Room 421
P.O. Box 8000
Old Westbury, New York 11568-8000
516-686-3883
www.nyit.edu/life_sciences/do
mharris@nyit.edu

SUNY New Paltz
1 Hawk Drive
NewPaltz, New York 12561
845-257-7869
www.newpaltz.edu/pre-health/nycom.html
admissions@newpaltz.edu

SUNY College at Old Westbury
P.O. Box 210
Old Westbury, New York 11568
516-876-3073
www.oldwestbury.edu/academics/offerings
/bsdo-osteopathic-medicine
enroll@oldwestbury.edu

NAME OF PROGRAM

B.S./D.O. Program

LENGTH OF PROGRAM

7 years

APPLICATION DEADLINE

December 15

INFORMATION ABOUT THE PROGRAM

No information provided.

TRANSFER STUDENTS CONSIDERED

No

CITIZENSHIP REQUIREMENTS

U.S. citizen or permanent resident visa

MINIMUM REQUIRED FACTORS IN SELECTION

CLASSES

No information provided

GPA

No information provided.

SAT

No information provided.

ACT

No information provided.

ACCEPTANCES

No information provided

FACTORS REQUIRED TO CONTINUE IN PROGRAM

No information provided

MCAT REQUIRED

No information provided

FINANCIAL AID

No special financial aid for students in the program

COST

	Resident Tuition and Fees ($)	Non Resident Tuition and Fees ($)
Undergraduate	Varies	Varies
Medical school	54,000	54,000

COLLEGE
Various Colleges

MEDICAL SCHOOL
Lake Erie College of Osteopathic Medicine

ADDRESS
1858 W. Grandview Boulevard
Erie, Pennsylvania 16509-1025
814-866-6641

20 Seton Hill Drive
Greensburg, Pennsylvania 15601
724-552-2880

5000 Lakewood Ranch Boulevard
Bradenton Florida 34211-4909
941-756-0690
http://lecom.edu/admissions/entrance-requirements
/early-acceptance-programs/

NAME OF PROGRAM
Early Acceptance Programs Admission Program

LENGTH OF PROGRAM
7 or 8 years

APPLICATION DEADLINE
Varies

INFORMATION ABOUT THE PROGRAM
LECOM has agreements with over 75 undergraduate schools. Students must apply to both LECOM and their undergraduate school of choice. The LECOM portion of the program can be completed on any of the three medical school campuses and students have the choice of a seven-year or eight-year program depending upon their choice of undergraduate school.

TRANSFER STUDENTS CONSIDERED
No

CITIZENSHIP REQUIREMENTS
U.S. citizen or permanent resident visa

MINIMUM REQUIRED FACTORS IN SELECTION

CLASSES
No information specified

GPA
3.5; 3.7 for seven-year track

SAT
1,170 math and critical reading; 1,250 math and critical reading for seven-year track

ACT
26; 28 for seven-year track

ACCEPTANCES
No information provided

FACTORS REQUIRED TO CONTINUE IN PROGRAM
Students must maintain an overall GPA of 3.4 and a science GPA of 3.2.

MCAT REQUIRED
Yes; must score above the national average

FINANCIAL AID
No special financial aid for students in the program

COST

	Resident Tuition and Fees ($)	Non Resident Tuition and Fees ($)
Undergraduate	Varies	Varies
Medical school	32,195	32,195

COLLEGE

Gannon University; University of the Sciences in Philadelphia

MEDICAL SCHOOL

Philadelphia College of Osteopathic Medicine

ADDRESS

Gannon University
Gitnik Manse
162 W. Sixth Street
Erie, Pennsylvania 16541
814-871-7240
www.gannon.edu/Academic-Offerings
/Health-Professions-and-Sciences/Undergraduate
/PCOM-Accelerated-Medical-Program/
admissions@gannon.edu

University of the Sciences in Philadelphia
600 South 43rd Street
Philadelphia, Pennsylvania 19104
215-596-8810
www.usciences.edu/academics/programs/premed/DualDegree
/PCOM.aspx
admit@usciences.edu

NAME OF PROGRAM

Dual Admission Program

LENGTH OF PROGRAM

7 or 8 years

APPLICATION DEADLINE

First come, first served basis

INFORMATION ABOUT THE PROGRAM

Students may major in any subject that results in obtaining a
BS. Students applying to the program should have three letters
of recommendation including one from a math or science teacher,
one from a humantities or social science teacher, and one from a
indivdual that can speak to the student's medical experiences. Finalists will be invited to interview at both the undergraduate and
medical school in February.

TRANSFER STUDENTS CONSIDERED

No

CITIZENSHIP REQUIREMENTS

U.S. citizen or permanent resident visa

MINIMUM REQUIRED FACTORS IN SELECTION

CLASSES

Students should have taken four years of English and math (through calculus), and three years of science including chemistry and physics.

GPA

3.4, top 25 percent of class

SAT

1,150 math and critical reading

ACT

25

ACCEPTANCES

A maximum of 5–10 students are accepted for this program per year from approximately 20 finalists.

FACTORS REQUIRED TO CONTINUE IN PROGRAM

Students must maintain an overall GPA of 3.5.

MCAT REQUIRED

Yes; must score above the national average

FINANCIAL AID

No special financial aid for students in the program

COST

	Resident Tuition and Fees ($)	Non Resident Tuition and Fees ($)
Undergraduate	48,400	48,400
Medical school	53,570	53,570

Index

A

ACT, 13–14, 33, 35
Activities résumé, 19–22, 54
Albany Medical College, 45–46,
 63–64, 152–157
American University of Antigua
 College of Medicine, 256–259
Augusta University, 102–103

B

Baylor College of Medicine, 47,
 230–237
Baylor University, 230–231
Boston University School of
 Medicine, 118–119
Brooklyn College, 158–159
Brown University, 7, 48, 62–63,
 77, 226–227
BS/DO program 32–33, 265–277

C

Caldwell College, 132–133,
 256–257, 260–261
California Northstate University,
 86–87
Case Western Reserve University
 School of Medicine, 186–187
Chadron State College, 128–129
Charles E. Schmidt College of
 Medicine, 98–99
Chicago College of Osteopathic
 Medicine- Midwestern
 University,
270–271
Clarkson University, 162–163

Clinical Skills, 28, 64
College of New Jersey, 134–135
Common Application, 19–21,
 36–41
CSS Profile, 70–71

D

doctor shadowing, *see* physician
 shadowing
Drexel University College of
 Medicine, 27, 47–48, 194–211
Drew University, 136–137

E

East Carolina University Brody
 School of Medicine, 182–185
essays
 undergraduate, 35–41
 medical school, 41–49
extracurriculars, 9, 17–22, 38

F

Feinberg School of Medicine, *see*
 Northwestern University
Florida Atlantic University, 98–99
Free Application for Federal
 Student Aid (FAFSA), 70-71, 74
Future Doctors of America, 18

G

Gannon University, 276–277
George Washington University
 School of Medicine and Health
 Sciences, 92–95

GPA, 6, 11–12, 30, 33, 62
Grambling State University,
    228–229
grants, 69–71, 74–75

H

Harvard Medical School, 75
Hobart and William Smith
    Colleges, 164–165
Hofstra University North Shore-
    LIJ School of Medicine,
    150–151
Howard University College of
    Medicine, 96–97

I

Illinois Institute of Technology,
    270–271
Indiana State University, 112–113
Indiana University School of
    Medicine
at Evansville, 114–115
at Terre Haute, 112–113
Inter American University of
    Puerto Rico at Ponce (UIA),
    222–223
international students, 77, 90,
    109, 118, 127, 181, 186, 212,
    227, 233, 262
interview, 6, 21–23, 49, 51–67

J

Jefferson Medical College,
    212–213
John A. Burns School of Medicine,
    see University of Hawai'i at
    Manoa

K

Kent State University, 188–189

L

Lake Erie College of Osteopathic
    Medicine (LECOM), 274–275
Lehigh University, 27, 196–197
loans, 69, 71, 73–75

M

Marshall University Joan C.
    Edwards School of Medicine,
    254–255
medical ethics, 45–46, 64–65
Medical College Admission Test
    (MCAT), 7, 10, 26–27, 63, 66
Medical College of Georgia,
    102–103
Meharry Medical College,
    228–229
Mercer University School of
    Medicine, 104–105
merit-based aid, 69–73
Miller School of Medicine, see
    University of Miami
Monmouth University, 198–199
Montclair State University,
    138–139
Muhlenberg College, 200–201

N

need-based aid, 69–73
New Jersey Institute of
    Technology, 140–141, 258–259,
    262–263
New York Institute of Technology,
    272–273
Northeast Ohio Medical
    University, 188–189
Northern Michigan University,
    120–121
Northwestern University, 4, 40,
    44, 77, 108–109
Nova Southeastern University,
    268–269

P

Penn State Hershey College of
    Medicine, 214–215
Penn State University, 47,
    212–213
Philadelphia College of
    Osteopathic Medicine, 276–277
physician shadowing, 16–17, 33,
    43, 59

Pitzer College, 266–267
Ponce School of Medicine, 222–225
Pontifical Catholic University of Puerto Rico (PUCPR), 224–225
Prairie View A & M University, 238–239, 248–249

R

recommendations, 22–23, 39
Rensselaer Polytechnic Institute, 64, 152–153
research experience, 14–15, 33, 39, 43–44, 58, 62
residency placement, 7, 9, 29, 33, 66
Rice University, 40, 47, 232–233
Richard Stockton College of New Jersey, 142–143
Robert Morris University, 202–203
Rosemont College, 204–205
Rutgers Biomedical and Health Sciences, 132–147
Rutgers-Newark College of Arts and Sciences, 144–145

S

SAT, 4, 13–14, 35
SAT subject test, 4, 14
scholarships, 7, 69–74
Siena College, 46, 154–155
St. Bonaventure University, 94–95, 166–167
St. George's University School of Medicine- Grenada, West Indies, 260–263
St. Lawrence University, 168–169
St. Mary's University, 246–247
State University of New York (SUNY) Health Science Center at Brooklyn, 158–159
Stevens Institute of Technology, 146–147
Stony Brook University School of Medicine, 160–161

South Texas College, 238–239
SUNY College of Environmental Science and Forestry, 170–171
SUNY Geneseo, 174–175
SUNY New Paltz, 272–273
SUNY Old Westbury, 272–273
SUNY Potsdam, 176–177
SUNY Upstate Medical University, 162–179
super-scoring, 13

T

Tarleton State University, 238–239
Temple University School of Medicine, 216–219
Texas A & M Health Science Center College of Medicine, 238–239
Texas A & M International University, 238–239, 246–249
Texas A & M University
    at College Station, 238–239
    at Commerce, 238–239
    at Corpus Christi, 2238–239
    at Kingsville, 238–239
Texas Southern University, 248–249
Texas Tech University- Health Sciences Center School of Medicine, 240–241
transferring, 31, 77–78, 125, 246

U

Union College, 45–46, 63, 156–157
United States Medical Licensing Exam (USMLE), 28–29, 32
University of Akron, 188–189
University of Alabama Birmingham, 30, 82–83
University of Cincinnati College of Medicine, 190–191
University of Colorado Denver School of Medicine, 88–89

University of Connecticut at
  Storrs School of Medicine, 48,
  90–91
University of Evansville, 114–115
University of Hawai'i at Manoa,
  106–107
University of Houston, 234–235
University of Illinois at Chicago
  College of Medicine, 110–111
University of Louisville School of
  Medicine, 116–117
University of Miami, 47, 100–101
University of Missouri Kansas
  City School of Medicine, 41,
  124–125
University of Nebraska Medical
  Center, 128–129
University of Nevada, Las Vegas,
  130–131
University of Nevada, Reno,
  130–131
University of New Mexico School
  of Medicine, 148–149
University of Oklahoma College of
  Medicine, 192–193
University of Pittsburgh School of
  Medicine, 220–221
University of Rochester School of
  Medicine, 46, 180–181
University of the Sciences in
  Philadelphia, 276–277
University of South Alabama
  College of Medicine, 84–85
University of Texas at
  Brownsville, see University of
  Texas at Rio Grande Valley
University of Texas at Dallas
  Southwestern Medical Center,
  244–245
University of Texas at El Paso,
  248–251
University of Texas Medical
  Branch at Galveston, 248–251
University of Texas Medical
  School-Houston, 250–251

University of Texas Pan
  American, 236–237, 246–247
University of Texas Pan American
  at Edinburg, 250–251
University of Texas at Rio Grande
  Valley, 236, 248–251
University of Texas at San
  Antonio Health Science Center,
  242–243, 246–247
Ursinus College, 206–207

V

Villanova University, 208–209
Virginia Commonwealth
  University School of Medicine,
  45, 252–253
volunteering, 9, 15–17, 19, 22, 30,
  33, 39, 46, 59

W

Warren Alpert Medical School, see
  Brown University
Washington & Jefferson College,
  218–219
Washington University in St.
  Louis School of Medicine, 30,
  126–127
Wayne State College, 128–129
Wayne State University School of
  Medicine, 120–123
West Chester University, 210–211
West Texas A & M University,
  238–239
Western University of Health
  Sciences, 266–267
Wilkes University, 178–179,
  214–215
work-study, 69, 71, 74

Y

Youngstown State University,
  188–189

For over a decade Todd Johnson has provided college admissions counseling to students throughout the United States. He has helped hundreds of students become the strongest candidates for BS/MD programs.

Todd is a graduate of St. Olaf College and the law school at Washington University in St. Louis, where he was the executive editor of the law review. Todd can be reached through his company website, www.collegeadmissionspartners.com.

■

Kelley Anne Johnson has worked with Todd Johnson, providing college admissions counseling to students applying to BS/MD programs. Kelley Anne is a graduate of Carleton College and obtained her Masters of Library and Information Science from the University of Illinois. She has worked in the fields of information and education throughout the United States and India.